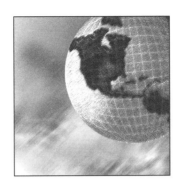

AIDS in the Modern World

I. Edward Alcamo, Ph.D.

Professor of Microbiology
State University of New York at Farmingdale

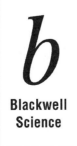

Blackwell Science

Editorial Offices:

Commerce Place, 350 Main Street,
    Malden, Massachusetts 02148, USA
Osney Mead, Oxford OX2 0EL, England
25 John Street, London WC1N 2BS, England
23 Ainslie Place, Edinburgh EH3 6AJ, Scotland
54 University Street, Carlton, Victoria 3053, Australia

Other Editorial Offices:

Blackwell Wissenschafts-Verlag GmbH,
    Kurfürstendamm 57, 10707 Berlin, Germany
Blackwell Science KK, MG Kodenmacho Building,
    7-10 Kodenmacho Nihombashi, Chuo-ku,
    Tokyo 104, Japan
Iowa State University Press,
    A Blackwell Science Company, 2121 S. State Avenue,
    Ames, Iowa 50014-8300, USA

Distributors:

The Americas

Blackwell Publishing
c/o AIDC
P.O. Box 20
50 Winter Sport Lane
Williston, VT 05495-0020
    (Telephone orders: 800-216-2522
    fax orders: 802-864-7626)

Australia

Blackwell Science Pty, Ltd.
54 University Street
Carlton, Victoria 3053
    (Telephone orders: 03-9347-0300;
    fax orders: 03-9349-3016)

Outside The Americas and Australia

Blackwell Science, Ltd.
c/o Marsten Book Services, Ltd.
P.O. Box 269
Abingdon
Oxon OX14 4YN
England
    (Telephone orders: 44-01235-465500;
    fax orders: 44-01235-465555)

Acquisitions: Nancy Whilton
Development: Jill Connor
Production: Shawn Girsberger
Manufacturing: Lisa Flanagan
Marketing Manager: Michael Rasmussen
Cover design by Leslie Haimes
Interior design by Leslie Haimes
Illustrations by Hans Neuhart, Electronic Illustrators Group
Typeset by Leslie Haimes
Printed and bound by Edwards Brothers, Inc.

Printed in the United States of America
02 03 04 05 5 4 3 2 1

Library of Congress Cataloging-in-Publication Data

Alcamo, I. Edward.
  AIDS in the modern world / I. Edward Alcamo.
    p. cm.
  ISBN 0-632-04474-8
  1. AIDS (Disease) I. Title.
  RC606.6 .A43 2001
  616.97'92—dc21
                                  2001001867

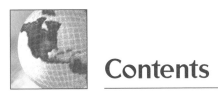

Contents

Preface

For an epidemic that would explode to claim hundreds of thousands of lives, AIDS surfaced very quietly in the United States. On June 4, 1981 in the weekly newsletter of the federal Centers For Disease Control and Prevention (CDC), public health officials alerted doctors to five unusual cases of pneumonia occurring in homosexual men in Los Angeles. The cases were unusual because all five men were well-nourished and vigorous until they became sick. And they had another thing in common—their immune systems had suffered a devastating loss of the T cells basic to the system. Without these cells, their immune systems had left their bodies acutely vulnerable to infectious disease, and the pneumonia that followed was lethal.

And so began the AIDS epidemic in the United States. In the years that followed, more and more cases would appear in sexually active homosexual men as well as injection drug users, patients with hemophilia, blood transfusion patients, heterosexuals, and children born to infected women. It soon became clear that the epidemic was shaped like an iceberg—for every person sick with AIDS, thousands more were infected with the virus responsible for the disease.

The AIDS epidemic would become the most serious public health problem of the last half of the 20th century. Today in the 21st century, much of the fear due to the epidemic has dissipated, in part because researchers have a good idea of what they are dealing with. For example, they know many details about the structure of the AIDS virus, how the virus is transmitted, how transmission can be interrupted, and what drugs can be used to slow its development in the body. They are familiar with how the virus affects the T cells, how AIDS manifests itself, and how a vaccine can be used to prevent the disease. These are but a few of the topics we shall consider in this book as we paint a picture of AIDS and the virus that causes it.

But the title of this book, *AIDS in the Modern World*, suggests a look at the current state of affairs of the AIDS epidemic. And so we shall highlight recent discoveries on how the AIDS virus attacks the immune system; we shall review the successful campaign to prevent AIDS in newborns; we shall explore the catastrophic effect of AIDS in Africa; we shall focus on the needle exchange programs that interrupt the spread of the AIDS virus; and we shall update the dramatic research in drug therapy that is encouraging AIDS patients to live longer and more fruitful lives. To be sure the progress has been slow; but it has also been steady.

AIDS in the Modern World is written for you, the mature lay reader. The objective is to present principles of the AIDS epidemic in a format that is easy to understand and comfortable to read. Biological concepts are intermixed with practical applications to bring you up-to-speed on the current status of the AIDS epidemic. It is hoped that on finishing this book, you will better comprehend the articles appearing in today's news media and thus become a more responsible and aware citizen. If you happen to think "Aha, that's what they mean!" then the mission of this book will have been fulfilled.

Using This Book

AIDS in the Modern World contains several strategies to help you learn the wealth of information relating to AIDS. One of the first things you will notice is that many of the passages are shaded in blue ink. These are key sentences of the chapter. Focusing on them will help you pick up the chapter's essential elements and make reviewing the chapter easier.

The chapters are organized like a progressive set of lectures, so each one begins with a Review and Preview. This section covers where we've been and gives a couple of thoughts on where we will be going in the chapter. It should prepare you to enter the chapter gracefully. In cases where you have read the chapters out of sequence, the Review and Preview sections should prepare you for that chapter's contents. They are somewhat like a "Last time on The West Wing…"

The science of AIDS is full of new and sometimes imposing terminology. To help you through, we've added the pronunciations of many of the terms. Knowing the pronunciations should make you more comfortable in using them and speaking about them. At the end of each chapter, there are three review questions that pull together some of the main points of the chapter. If you can answer them confidently, then you have mastered some of the chapter's key thoughts.

Acknowledgements

I am pleased to acknowledge the contributions of several valued professionals to the completion of this work. Among the reviewers were Donald Emmeluth of Armstrong Atlantic State University, Thomas Budd of St. Lawrence University, David Kelly of George Mason University, Vincent Lynch of Boston College, and Leland Russell of St. Edward's College. At Blackwell Science, Nancy Whilton supervised the project with a careful and discerning eye; and Shawn Girsberger used her considerable talents to guide the production process through its usual highs and lows. The manuscript was expertly copyedited by Vickie West; the photos were tracked down by Billie Porter; and Karen Bonura typed the manuscript with a knowledgeable touch. I thank each of them collectively.

I also received wonderful support from my family. My loving wife Charlene was there to push me along when I needed a gentle nudge and to share moments of success when things came into focus. And our children Michael, Elizabeth, Tracey, and Patricia shared their love and affection, while encouraging me to assume the sometimes lonely task of writing.

Finally I acknowledge you the reader who has picked up this book. Thanks for spending some time with it and for your interest in one of the key health issues of our times. Best wishes for a successful learning experience.

I. E. Alcamo
Summer, 2001

Chapter One

The Emergence of AIDS

Preview

Medical historians will report that AIDS has been one of the great challenges confronting public health during the 20th and 21st centuries. More than any other disease, AIDS affects all segments of society: young and old, rich and poor, black and white. Stories about AIDS permeate the news media like no other disease of this generation, and they will continue to do so until an effective preventive or complete cure is found.

In this chapter, we introduce acquired immune deficiency syndrome, or as it is better known, AIDS. We will examine how AIDS emerged in society, where it currently is centered, and where it may be going. The first observations were made in 1980, when a patient exhibited a then-obscure, ill-defined disease. From that case onward, physicians believed that something new had appeared on the medical landscape and that it was of serious nature.

As the epidemic continued to spread in society, scientists came to the realization that it was affecting broad segments of the national and international populations, and they focused their attention on isolating the cause. As we shall see, they could find nothing to explain the disease; during the first few years of the epidemic, it was a disease without a cause. However, it had a name: AIDS.

When a virus was finally isolated in 1984, scientists identified it as the cause of the new epidemic. Now it was possible to develop a diagnostic test and begin the search for therapeutic drugs and vaccines. Soon the attitude toward the disease shifted from viewing AIDS as an acute plague to regarding it as a chronic disease. The discovery of a useful and effective drug, AZT, encouraged this new perspective.

Now, the original "AIDS" is recognized as two diseases: HIV infection and AIDS. We will discuss the difference between the two conditions, both of which can be caused by different strains of human immunodeficiency virus (HIV). This chapter also presents some recent statistics regarding the AIDS epidemic, which illustrate its spread throughout the world. Since the beginning of the epidemic, scientists have wondered about its origin and the origin of HIV. The current evidence points to an African primate as the source. And finally, to close the chapter, we will examine the ideas of Paul Ewald, an evolutionary biologist who believes that behavioral changes are a key to interrupting the epidemic's spread. The concepts presented in this chapter set the foundation for the fuller discussion of AIDS in the chapters ahead.

Introduction

In the fall of 1980, a resident physician at the UCLA Medical Center was visited by a 31-year-old patient suffering from persistent fever, weight loss, and swollen lymph nodes. The patient, a sexually active homosexual male, also had a severe yeast infection in his mouth and throat. Yeasts are single-celled fungi often found in the body, which usually cause no harm. The yeast infection, known as candidiasis (kan"-di-di'ah-sis), is often observed in patients undergoing chemotherapy for cancer. It also occurs in individuals whose immune systems are depressed, such as those who have had transplant surgery.

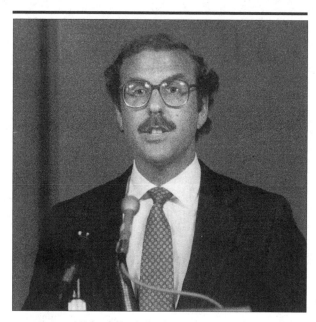

FIGURE 1.1 Michael Gottlieb, the UCLA internist whose observations of immunodeficient patients in 1980 opened the investigation to the newly emerging disease that would later be named AIDS.

The resident brought the patient to the attention of Michael Gottlieb, an internist at UCLA. Gottlieb, pictured in Figure 1.1, noted that the patient had a lung infection as well as the yeast infection, and he obtained samples of the patient's lung fluid and sent them to the lab, where technologists observed a protozoan named *Pneumocystis carinii* (new"mo-sis'tis car-in'e-e). This organism is known to cause a rare type of pneumonia referred to as *Pneumocystis* pneumonia. In most cases, the disease occurs in individuals who are suffering from a deficiency of immune system functions. In a healthy person, the protozoa are readily eliminated by cells of the immune system called T cells (technically known as T lymphocytes). When Gottlieb examined tissue from the immune system of his patient, he observed that an entire subgroup of T cells known as helper T cells had been largely destroyed. He and his colleagues were mildly dumbfounded—nothing in the medical literature seemed to address their observation.

Then, in February 1981, Gottlieb was presented with

another patient suffering the same combination of yeast and protozoal infections. This patient also had Kaposi's (kap'o-seez) sarcoma, a very rare skin neoplasm primarily found in older men of Mediterranean descent and individuals with depressed immune systems. The new patient, another sexually active homosexual male, also had a depleted content of helper T cells.

By April of that year, four additional cases had come to Gottlieb's attention. The common feature among all patients was their homosexuality and their participation in anal sex. Gottlieb wrote a brief report to the Federal Centers for Disease Control and Prevention (CDC), an agency of the U.S. Public Health Service concerned with the investigation and prevention of epidemics. It reported Gottlieb's account on June 1981 in its weekly newsletter of public health issues *Morbidity and Mortality Weekly Reports*. This was the first public report concerning the disease that would one day be called acquired immune deficiency syndrome (AIDS). The publication of this report is regarded as the beginning of the AIDS epidemic.

One physician receiving the public health newsletter was Willy Rozenbaum of the Claude Bernard Hospital in Paris. Rozenbaum responded that three years earlier he had also treated a man suffering from *Pneumocystis* pneumonia. His patient had recently arrived from Africa. And two years earlier he had treated two women from Africa, both with *Pneumocystis* pneumonia. In the interim, all three patients had died. It appeared that the same malady affecting the homosexual men in Los Angeles was also infecting Rozenbaum's African patients.

Rozenbaum, Gottlieb, and their colleagues were perplexed as to the cause of the illnesses. Rozenbaum was inclined to believe the disease was caused by an infectious agent because it appeared to be transmissible. Because several years had passed between the observations in Paris and Los Angeles, he suggested that the disease had been in the human population for some time and that it had a very long incubation period (the incubation period is the time passing between entry of an infectious agent and the appearance of symptoms.) The implications were that the disease could take hold in the world's population long before evidence of its presence was detected.

The Early Observations

Epidemiologists, the first scientists to investigate the mysterious new ailment, were struck by its seeming preference for young, homosexual males. The scientists searched for causes in the behaviors common to gay men, including risk factors prevalent in this group such as anal sex and use of the drug amyl nitrate. The disease soon came to be called by the disparaging name GRID, meaning gay-related immune disease. But soon the disease was also observed in distinctly different groups in the United States, such as male and female injection drug users, and blood transfusion recipients.

As the months passed, female sex partners of bisexual

men and injection drug users began showing signs of the disease. Infants born to infected mothers or women with a history of injection drug use also displayed the disease. In 1983, a study found that hemophiliacs with no history of any proposed causes of the disease were developing the syndrome, and some men had apparently transmitted the infection to their wives. Early suspects as the disease's cause were cytomegalovirus (si"to-meg'a-lo-virus) because of its association with immune suppression, and Epstein-Barr virus, which has an attraction for lymphocytes. However, studies of blood sera failed to show convincing evidence that these viruses had a primary role in the syndrome.

By 1982, the new disease had received a permanent name: acquired immune deficiency syndrome, or AIDS. The term was first used by researcher Bruce R. Voeller, who coined the term as a protest to the disease's earlier label of GRID. The CDC soon introduced the term in its weekly public health report. From 1961 to 1972, Voeller was on the faculty of Rockefeller University. He was a co-founder of the National Gay Task Force and served as its executive director for many years. The name AIDS reflected the ability of the disease to be transmitted, the involvement of the immune system, and the understanding at that time that it was a collection of symptoms (a syndrome), rather than a defined disease with a known agent.

AIDS As an Infectious Disease

In 1983, researchers provided the first evidence linking AIDS to a certain type of virus called a retrovirus (Chapter 2). Then, in April 1983, the AIDS virus was isolated and cultivated by Luc Montagnier (Figure 1.2A) and a group of French investigators at the Pasteur Institute in Paris. Simultaneously, Robert Gallo (Figure 1.2B) and a group of American researchers also isolated the virus, using tissue samples that had been sent to him by Montagnier. For the first two years, the virus was called lymphadenopathy virus (LAV), as well as human T-lymphotropic virus III (HTLV-III). In 1986 it received the name human immunodeficiency virus (HIV). By that time, the number of cases of AIDS had swelled to over 25,000 individuals and the number of deaths to over 13,000.

During the 1980s, examination of sera collected in association with hepatitis B studies suggested that HIV had entered the U.S. population sometime in the late-1970s. Another study showed that 4.5 percent of men in San Francisco who had hepatitis B also had antibodies to HIV. (Antibodies are defensive proteins produced by the body's immune system when confronted by a foreign organism.) Moreover, research indicated that in 1978, at least one batch of Factor VIII used to treat hemophilia patients was contaminated with HIV. Factor VIII was given to over 2000 hemophiliac males in the United States that year. By July 1982, the first cases of AIDS in hemophiliac patients were reported.

In 1984, the identification of the human immunodeficiency virus (HIV) as the cause of AIDS opened to a new phase in which AIDS was characterized as an infectious disease. Scientists could now use laboratory studies of the virus and determine its action within the body, hoping to make new discoveries leading to treatments and vaccines. Identification of HIV also focused popular views on the causes of the AIDS epidemic, because people had a familiar, if vague, understanding of a virus. Because a virus was perceived as something easy to "catch," many well-informed people began to fear contact with

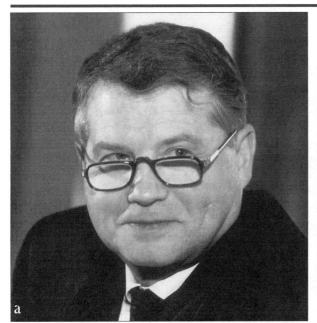
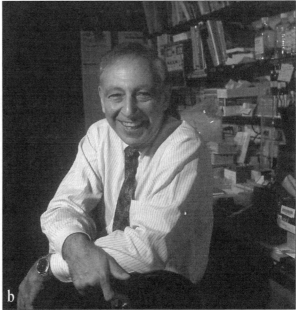

FIGURE 1.2 The HIV discoverers. (a) Luc Montagnier, the French researcher who was the first to isolate and cultivate HIV. (b) Robert Gallo, the American investigator who simultaneously isolated the same virus from samples sent him by Montagnier.

AIDS patients. Among health professionals, the identification of HIV clarified strategies for AIDS prevention.

The identification of the virus also shifted attention away from risk-group designations (e.g., homosexual males), and instead highlighted the importance of risk behaviors and acts (e.g., high risk sexual practices). Public health professionals now advocated practical, simple, and individual-oriented methods of prevention, such as using condoms to help block HIV transmission. For injection drug users, clean needles were recommended. Ultimately the identification of HIV and the development of a blood test encouraged a traditional approach to controlling an epidemic: identify infected individuals and isolate them to interrupt transmission.

An important attitude change occurred in the late 1980s when scientists began thinking of AIDS not as a plague but as a chronic disease. One reason was that the epidemic was developing over a lengthy period of time and was not disappearing quickly. This pattern contrasted sharply with the epidemics of smallpox, typhoid fever, cholera, and the other great "slate-wipers" of history. Also, statisticians were noting reduced estimates of the number of persons infected with HIV. And infected individuals were living longer than individuals lived during the traditional epidemics. Thus, the emphasis was changing from "dying from AIDS" to "living with AIDS."

Also during the late 1980s, although the research continued to focus on prevention, it had expanded to include potential therapies and vaccine development. The development of treatments such as azidothymidine (az-i-doh-thy'mi-deen) placed new emphasis on therapy. This drug is best known by its acronym AZT and by its alternate name of zidovudine (zy-doh'vu-deen), or ZDV. Soon the health services and the number of dedicated AIDS units for inpatient and outpatient care were increasing. Even the image of AIDS as an unmanageable financial burden on society began to disappear. As a chronic disease, AIDS was soon being compared to tuberculosis, cancer, and cardiovascular disease. All are debilitating and often fatal conditions that are slow to develop, persist for many years, and require long-term management. Screening, early detection, and treatment are essential to the management of such diseases.

Development of the Epidemic

Blood tests to detect HIV carriers were made available in 1985, and for the first time people could be tested to see if they were at risk for developing AIDS. Scientists could also get some idea of the epidemic's form and guess how it might develop further. It was clear that the epidemic resembled an iceberg: It had a small, visible tip with a huge invisible base; that is, for every person sick with AIDS, thousands of others were infected with HIV but showed no symptoms yet. Often they were not even aware that they were infected. Although these individuals had "HIV infection," not AIDS, they were still able to transmit the virus to others, a factor that encouraged the spread of

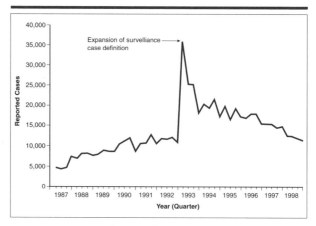

FIGURE 1.3 Reported cases of AIDS in the United States from 1987 to 1998. Note that when the case definition of AIDS was revised in 1993, the number of cases rose dramatically because more individuals were now considered AIDS patients. Since that time, the number of cases has continued its overall decline.

the epidemic. The medical jargon for such individuals is "HIV-positive."

By the end of 1988, almost 90,000 Americans had been diagnosed with AIDS and over 50,000 had died. At that time, public health officials estimated that close to a million might be carrying the virus in the United States and have HIV infection, although the epidemic was slowing in the United States, as Figure 1.3 shows. By 1995, almost a half million Americans had been diagnosed with AIDS and over half had died. AZT, the first useful drug shown to have anti-HIV activity, was in use. Unfortunately, it had many side effects; and it failed to prevent healthy people from becoming ill and developing AIDS. Nevertheless, it was used to prevent HIV from passing from mother to child during pregnancy, and the number of infected newborns began to decline thereafter. By 1996 a new class of drugs called protease inhibitors were in use. These drugs are discussed in Chapter 9.

Toward the end of the 1980s, a second major strain of HIV was identified. Labeled HIV-2, the strain was found to exist primarily in West Africa. Physicians determined that it was a less lethal strain than HIV-1. Both HIV-1 and HIV-2 are genetically similar to viruses found in African primates. These viruses are called simian immunodeficiency viruses or SIVs. HIV-2 is quite similar to the SIV that infects the sooty mangabey, an ash-colored monkey. Indeed, some researchers believe that the mangabey virus is nearly identical to HIV-2, as we discuss later in this chapter.

Recent Statistics

In late 1999, the Centers for Disease Control and Prevention announced that deaths from AIDS were decreasing steadily. For example, in 1996 there were 37,221 deaths associated with AIDS, but only 21,445 in 1997 and 17,171 in 1998. These sta-

TABLE 1.1   Estimated Deaths of Persons with AIDS, Grouped by Year of Death and Region of Residence in the United States

Region of Residence	Year of Death					
	1993	**1994**	**1995**	**1996**	**1997**	**1998**
Northeast	13,984	15,858	15,768	11,514	6,670	4,950
Midwest	4,767	5,186	5,420	4,005	2,277	1,800
South	14,411	16,063	16,951	13,440	8,186	7,026
West	10,274	10,579	10,071	6,719	3,342	2,651
U.S. dependencies, possessions, and associated nations	1,555	1,757	1,685	1,543	970	744
Total	**44,991**	**49,442**	**49,895**	**37,221**	**21,445**	**17,171**

tistics are shown in Table 1.1, organized by region of the United States. In addition, in 1996 AIDS was not one of the top 10 causes of death for the first time since 1991. Accidents displaced AIDS as the leading cause of death in adult individuals 25 to 44 years old. However, at the beginning of the 21st century the infection rate has been holding steady at about 40,000 new cases per year; in some poor communities, the rate is increasing. Part of the reason is the cost of drug therapy. Use of the new drugs can cost more than $10,000 per year. In June 2000, the CDC reported that there had been 745,103 cases of AIDS since the beginning of the epidemic and 438,795 deaths associated with the disease.

At the current time doctors predict that many persons with AIDS may live and thrive for many years. In this sense AIDS has become a chronic disease. It has been found in recent years, however, that HIV has hundreds of different strains and can mutate easily. Also, it can develop resistance to drugs in a relatively short period of time. Moreover, the AIDS treatments are extremely expensive and are not available in impoverished countries of Africa and Asia. Unfortunately, the vast majority of the world's HIV-positive population lives on these continents.

At present, the best hope against AIDS lies in the development of a vaccine, but there are numerous problems attending this development, as we shall see in other chapters. Until an effective vaccine is available, the best methods for prevention include education, encouraging people to be tested, and developing effective methods for discouraging drug use and encouraging condom use.

The Current AIDS Pandemic

A pandemic is a global epidemic. In 2000, about 35 million people worldwide were living with HIV infection and/or AIDS. Of that 35 million, about 5 million became infected that year. According to public health agencies, the epidemic is expanding, with an estimated doubling time of 10 years; AIDS has now surpassed tuberculosis and malaria as the leading cause of death from an infectious disease in the world.

During 1999, about 2.6 million people worldwide died of AIDS and its effects. Nearly 70 percent of the new infections occurred in sub-Saharan Africa, which continues to be the hardest hit region on the globe. In several African countries, more than one-fifth of the adult population is HIV-positive.

Even in the United States where the death rate from AIDS is declining because of effective drug therapy, the infection rate of HIV continues to climb in women and members of racial and ethnic minorities. To address this public health crisis, the National Institutes of Health (NIH) is expanding its program of HIV prevention research. The aim of the NIH is to develop interventions for protecting uninfected people and for reducing the risk of transmission by sexual, bloodborne, or prenatal routes. Behavioral and social interventions include reducing the number of an individual's sex partners, delaying the age of initiation to sexual activity, reducing the incidence of sexually transmitted diseases, directing injection drug users to drug treatment programs, reducing needle sharing, and reducing the frequency of drug injection. These interventions are particularly important because the estimated number of persons living with AIDS continues to grow, as Table 1.2 illustrates. In minority groups the growth is insidious.

The Origin of HIV

Viruses are the ultimate parasites. Unlike bacteria, which absorb nutrients, excrete wastes, and reproduce by dividing, viruses have no life of their own. They are particles of genetic information (encoded in DNA or RNA), with a surrounding capsule of protein and, in some cases, an enclosing membranous envelope. They integrate themselves into a living cell and use its biochemical machinery to produce copies of themselves, as the next chapter will explore. The origin of viruses is unknown, but modern viruses are descendants of earlier forms.

There are several popular theories having to do with the origin of HIV and the AIDS epidemic. Among them is a conspiracy theory indicating that HIV was produced by a terrorist

TABLE 1.2   Estimated Persons Living with AIDS, Grouped by Year and Race/Ethnic Group

Race/Ethnicity	Year					
	1993	1994	1995	1996	1997	1998
White, not Hispanic	80,582	86,999	92,172	99,202	108,031	116,445
Black, not Hispanic	60,752	72,029	81,489	92,540	105,719	118,525
Hispanic	31,241	36,579	41,169	46,371	52,455	58,185
Asian/Pacific Islander	1,284	1,447	1,606	1,849	2,088	2,320
American Indian/Alaska Native	559	657	710	796	890	971
Total	174,633	197,986	217,508	241,221	269,775	297,136

researcher using a hybrid virus engineered from other retro-viruses. Most scientists see this as nonsense.

Another questionable theory is that HIV was an unfortunate side effect of polio vaccination campaigns carried out in the then-Belgian Congo in the late 1950s. Propagated in 1992, the story purports to show that through a complex process, HIV arose from monkey and ape cells used in the oral polio vaccine production. However, a blue-ribbon panel of scientists convened in 1993 indicated that almost every step in this hypothetical mode of transmission is difficult to believe. Indeed, the scientist named as director of the polio vaccine project (and "contaminator of the vaccine") sued the magazine first reporting the story and won a substantial settlement for defamation of character. And in 1999, the book *The River* detailed the hypothesis further, and a meeting sponsored by the Royal Society addressed all aspects of the oral polio vaccine hypothesis. The hypothesis has now been ruled implausible.

For many years, scientists agreed that the human immunodeficiency viruses were probably derived from ape or monkey viruses. Then, in 1999, Beatrice Hahn of the University of Alabama at Birmingham announced her research findings confirming what scientists had long suspected: HIV-1 came from African chimpanzees. Hahn traced the virus to a subspecies of chimpanzee called *Pan troglodytes* (tro-glo-di'tes). Hahn and her team fit the human and chimpanzee viruses into genetic "family trees" accounting for the similarities and differences. They showed that the chimpanzee viruses most closely related to HIV-1 exist in West Central Africa, the same region where all known variants of HIV-1 are found and where the greatest diversity of the main form of HIV-1 has been found.

As part of her research, Hahn obtained tissue samples taken in 1985 from a healthy chimpanzee caught in the wild in the area of study and who died at a U.S. primate facility after giving birth to stillborn twins. She amplified the genome of unknown virus from the animal's lymph node. Since this discovery, a research team at the Pasteur Institute has discovered three additional viruses from West Central African chimpanzees. Hahn has concluded that West Central African chimpanzees were the natural host and reservoir for existing HIV-1 strains. It is unclear whether chimpanzees continue to serve as reservoirs for the virus.

In addition, the researchers suggested a plausible mode of transmission from chimpanzee to humans: chimpanzees were long hunted for food, and blood from the animal's carcass may have entered the hunter's body through a superficial wound. Hahn's group showed how, after jumping species on at least three occasions, the chimpanzee virus evolved into the three families of HIV-1 recognized today. They noted that the chimpanzees carrying the virus do not appear to get sick from it, which could reveal important clues about controlling AIDS. The genes of chimpanzees are 98.5 percent similar to human genes. Therefore, studying the virus-animal interactions may give insight as to why the chimpanzee seems to be resistant to the disease.

Also, in 1999 researchers led by David Ho announced that they had isolated fragments of the HIV virus from a blood sample drawn in 1959 from a man living in what was then the Belgian Congo (now Democratic Republic of Congo). By comparing genetic sequences of these segments with sequences from more recent strains of HIV, they created a family tree and traced elements in the 1959 sample to a common ancestor of three present-day subtypes of HIV-1. The 1959 virus closely resembles ancestral virus believed to have passed from its animal host (chimpanzee) into humans. The researchers suspect that the passage occurred in the late 1950s or mid-1940s. The movements of peoples, the introduction of motor cars, and/or the disruptions and migrations in post-colonial Africa may have played a key role in the spread of HIV.

The prevailing theory holds that humans were first infected via direct contact with primates. The theory continues that the SIV then diverged from its ancestors and gave rise to the current form. It is possible, of course, that humans were the original carriers, but the primate-to-human scenario is favored over the human-to-primate scenario for two reasons. First, SIVs are more varied than HIVs, which suggests they have been evolving for a longer period of time. Second, it is more reasonable to imagine that humans have been infected by chimpanzees or monkeys than vice versa. This is because humans have hunted and handled other primates for thousands of years, and a bite or scratch or cut sustained while butchering an animal could account for transmission.

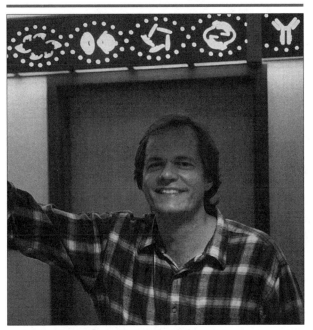

FIGURE 1.4 Contemporary AIDS researcher Paul Ewald, whose theory points to the spread of HIV as a function of social changes occurring in the world.

The Effects of Social Change

Paul Ewald, an evolutionary biologist from Amherst College, argues that HIV may have infected people for decades without causing disease. He traces the virulence of HIV to the social upheavals of the 1960s and 1970s, which not only sped the movement of HIV through populations but rewarded it for reproducing more aggressively within the body. Ewald (see Figure 1.4) suggests that, to pass between individuals, HIV particles are sequestered within the T cells they infect. These cells pass only during the exchange of body fluids or during sexual intercourse. When confined to an isolated population in which a carrier lacks sex partners, a virus such as HIV gains little from replicating aggressively. The virus "allows" the host to remain alive and the virus remains mildly infectious. However, if the carrier has numerous sex partners, fresh hosts are plentiful, and the infected hosts are more dispensable. An HIV strain might replicate wildly under these circumstances and kill people in a relatively short period of time.

Such social changes occurred in the 1960s. The outside world entered into Africa's once-isolated villages through war and tourism. Drought, industrialization, and civil wars prompted mass migrations from the countryside into the cities, and urbanization shattered the normal social structures constraining sexual behavior. Prostitution and sexually transmitted diseases flourished, and hypodermic needles came into widespread use with the creation of the drug culture. During these times a chronic but relatively benign infection may have become a killer.

Ewald's ideas suggest that HIV assumes different personalities in different settings. The virus is more aggressive when it is traveling rapidly through a population and more benign in stable and isolated groups. This conclusion is enhanced by the observation that HIV-2 is mild in the stable and isolated West African nations, whereas HIV-1 is a rapidly spreading virus and is responsible for most cases of AIDS in the United States. West Africa escaped much of the war, drought, and urbanization that fueled the spread of HIV-1 in the central and eastern parts of that continent.

A natural offshoot of Ewald's theory is that combating AIDS can be performed adequately by applying pressures to prevent transmission. For example, condoms and clean needles save lives by preventing HIV passage. These implements also push the virus toward more benevolent forms because they deprive the virulent strains of the high transmission rates they need to survive. Safer sex practices may encourage HIV to become less virulent, and other prevention efforts could conceivably convert the virulence of HIV-1 into the relatively benign virulence showed by HIV-2.

Not coincidentally, these recommendations coincide with those of public health officials. Ultimately, the AIDS epidemic may come to an end not because of drugs or vaccines, but because of preventative measures and behavioral changes. We shall see how these are implemented in the chapters ahead.

Questions

1. Discuss some of the events surrounding the first observations of the human immunodeficiency virus (HIV) in humans.

2. Summarize the evidence that led scientists to conclude that HIV is transmissible among humans by contaminated blood and body fluids.

3. Explain the currently accepted theory for the appearance of HIV in human populations.

Chapter Two

HIV and Human Disease

Review and Preview

In Chapter 1, we set the stage, for this chapter by discussing the origin and first observations of AIDS. We showed how scientists had been initially mystified about the new ailment in the American population, and how they found that numerous groups could be afflicted. Researchers focused on blood as a means of transmission because those who were developing the disease had some history of receiving blood. They also discovered that semen could transmit the virus, so they researched possible modes of sexual transmission. For the first two years of the epidemic, the disease had no name; by 1982, the term *acquired immunodeficiency syndrome* (AIDS) had been coined and was in use in public health agencies, though it had not yet been adopted by the general public.

Discovery of the human immunodeficiency virus (HIV) was a major breakthrough in AIDS research, and credit for the discovery is attributed to a French research group led by Luc Montagnier. Once a virus was identified, scientists could look for evidence of HIV in blood samples from patients, and they soon came to understand the global impact of the epidemic. Furthermore, they could now hunt for anti-HIV drugs, and the identification of azidothymidine (AZT) as a useful therapy began the period in which AIDS became less an acute disease and more a chronic disease, one that could be managed like tuberculosis, diabetes, and certain cancers.

As AIDS continued to spread, it took a heavy toll on the American and international populations, and a second strain of HIV was identified in Africa. Toward the late 1990s, the death rate in the United States decreased because of the use of AZT combined with a new class of drugs called protease inhibitors. However, these drugs are not available worldwide,

and globally, about 30 million people continue to live with HIV infection and/or AIDS. Behavioral and social interventions are key considerations in delaying the spread of the epidemic.

Since the discovery of HIV in 1984, scientists have investigated its origins. Various sources were postulated, but research in 1999 pointed to an African primate, a subspecies of chimpanzee, as the source of the virus. Also that year, scientists showed that HIV was present in a blood sample that had been drawn in 1959, which indicates that the epidemic was well underway before it was identified in the United States in 1981.

In Chapter 2 we begin the in-depth examination of AIDS by focusing on two important concepts: how disease works and how the body mounts resistance to disease. It is important to understand the basis for infectious disease so that we can fit AIDS into the pattern. It is equally important that we understand how the immune system works because it is the target of infection by HIV. By destroying the body's capability of mounting a defense, HIV leaves the body susceptible for infection by other microbes. This is a key to understanding AIDS.

In this presentation we shall look at the disease process and some of the factors that contribute to disease. These include dose, adherence, the interaction of viruses with cells, and the destruction of cells by viruses. We shall also explain some of the medical concepts used to describe various kinds of disease so that we can discuss AIDS effectively. Once we have established the foundations for disease and immunity, then we can discuss how AIDS brings about its profound changes. These discussions will follow in future presentations.

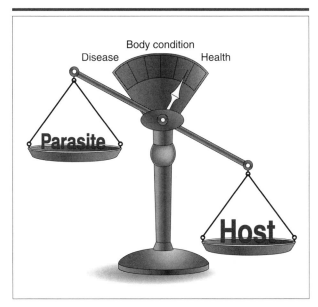

FIGURE 2.1 The balance between health and disease as it takes place in the human body.

Introduction

Infectious disease is a profound human experience: A population of organisms, invisible to the unaided eye, gain entry to the body, multiply in its tissues, and bring about a change from good health. Infectious disease results from a competition between the microorganism and the host, a competition that often leads to illness and, in some cases, death. Figure 2.1 illustrates this principle.

Under normal conditions, the body is continually "infected." It contains a normal flora, the population of microorganisms in the mouth and gastrointestinal tract, on every inch of its skin, and virtually anywhere that the body contacts the environment. Most of the time, the microorganisms live in a harmonious relationship with the body, sometimes providing nutrients or keeping disease-causing organisms under control. But within this normal flora are opportunists, organisms that wait for the opportunity to infect the tissues, such as when the immune system is depressed as happens in an individual with AIDS. In other cases, microorganisms with unusual abilities happen along. These organisms, known as pathogens, invariably induce infectious disease. HIV is a pathogen because it penetrates body cells and multiplies within them.

Pathogenicity

The capacity of a microbe to bring about disease is known as pathogenicity. Pathogenicity refers to the ability of a microorganism to invade a host and avoid its defenses while multiplying in and destroying its tissues. Some bacteria produce extremely powerful toxins that poison body cells and tissues, while other microbes such as HIV overwhelm the body cells with their extraordinary numbers. These pathogens stand in stark contrast to microbes such as fermentation yeasts, which have little or no pathogenic capacity.

To respond to disease, the human body possesses various mechanisms of resistance. Some mechanisms are continually in operation. (An example is the phagocytosis performed by microbe-engulfing white blood cells.) Other defenses such as antibodies are produced only in response to the presence of a microorganism. How well these responses perform will largely determine whether the body returns to good health.

The Disease Process

Infectious disease is a complex series of interactions between microbe and host, and depending upon which prevails, the disease will take different courses. Microorganisms enter the body by various modes, including skin penetration at a wound site, ingestion with food, inhalation as aerosols, or contact with objects such as kitchen utensils. Where a microbe enters the body can be an important factor, because some species can only survive in certain locations in the body. For example, *Salmonella* species will cause intestinal infection if they enter via food, but they usually will not cause a skin infection if they contact the skin. Moreover, the human immunodeficiency virus (HIV) will thrive in cells of the immune system, but not on the skin or within the gastrointestinal tract.

Another consideration is dose. This concept implies that a certain threshold number of pathogens must be present to establish infection. For *Salmonella* infections in the intestine, the dose level may be as low as several hundred bacilli, but for cholera it may be several million bacilli. The reason for this disparity is that most cholera bacilli are destroyed by the stomach acid, but *Salmonella* cells are acid-resistant. For AIDS to develop in the body, a substantial number of HIV particles must penetrate the body surface into the blood. This is why an exposure to contaminated blood or semen must be significant—merely touching a drop of blood with intact skin will probably not result in transmission of HIV.

Adherence to the host cell's surface will also enhance the virulence of an organism because attachment encourages colonization at the infection site or permits penetration to the cell's interior. Figure 2.2 displays an example of adherence. As we shall see, HIV possesses on its surface the necessary proteins that encourage it to interact with the T cells of the body's immune system and initiate the disease process. The virus possesses the molecular key that fits into the cellular lock at the beginning of the infection cycle. In many cases, viruses bring about disease by destroying the cells in which they multiply during their process of replication, as Chapter 3 discusses. The human immunodeficiency virus is a notable example because it multiplies in the body's T cells and gradually eliminates them. In so doing, it considerably lowers the body's

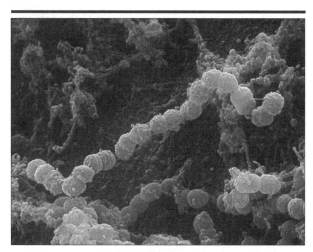

FIGURE 2.2 An electron micrograph of microorganisms adhering at a tissue site. Adherence is an important factor in the establishment of infectious disease.

ability to fight off opportunistic microbes.

Viruses can destroy cells by other means as well. Certain viruses kill by inducing cells to release enzymes from their lysosomes, a series of submicroscopic bodies in the cell's cytoplasm. In still other cases, viruses force themselves through the cell's membrane (they "bud" through) at the conclusion of the replication cycle, thereby puncturing holes in the membrane. If these holes cannot be repaired in time, the cells leak their cytoplasm and disintegrate. This is a way that HIV can kill T cells.

 ## Concepts of Infectious Disease

As the competition between the pathogen and host continues, a certain recognizable pattern exists in the progress of the disease. Initially, there is a period of incubation, reflecting the time between the pathogen's entry into the host and the appearance of symptoms. In HIV infection and AIDS, this period tends to be extremely long. Next comes the period of prodromal symptoms, a time when nonspecific symptoms such as nausea, fever, lymph node swelling, and other evidences of disease prevail. This period occurs during HIV infection. Then comes the period of acme, or height of disease, when specific symptoms such as severe cellular destruction develop in the patient. Now the patient with HIV infection has progressed to AIDS. Opportunistic illnesses, the diseases caused by opportunistic organisms, are frequent during this period.

Infectious diseases may be acute or chronic. An acute disease develops rapidly and runs its course quickly; a chronic disease develops more slowly and persists for a long period of time. An illness such as influenza is considered acute, but one such as AIDS is usually considered chronic. Moreover, a disease can be local when confined to a specific area of the body, or systemic when it spreads to other parts of the body. AIDS

occurs in T cells found in lymph nodes throughout the body, so it is a systemic disease.

Disease can occur in a localized or widespread area. Diseases found at a low level within a restricted population are known as endemic diseases. Diseases that occur explosively within a population are said to be epidemic. (Influenza epidemics are a well-known example.) A worldwide epidemic is referred to as a pandemic. During the early years, AIDS was considered an epidemic, but as the disease spread, it came to be known as a pandemic. Thus, public health officials now speak of the "AIDS pandemic."

To deal with the formidable challenge of infectious disease, the human body possesses a number of defensive mechanisms classified as nonspecific and specific. Nonspecific mechanisms involve a broad series of factors such as chemical and mechanical barriers and nonspecific substances. Specific forms of immunity involve the immune system, one of the principal body systems. We shall briefly note the first mechanism, then we will concentrate on the immune system as we discuss the body's answer to the microbe's challenge.

Nonspecific Resistance

Nonspecific resistance exists in all humans and is present from the earliest time of life. It protects against all microbes, regardless of their nature. Nonspecific defenses constitute the body's first line of defense against disease.

Included in the nonspecific defenses of the body are the anatomical barriers such as the skin and mucous membranes. The skin's epidermis has several layers of cells filled with a waterproofing protein known as keratin. HIV penetrates these layers when a person having skin cuts, scratches, or lesions makes contact with HIV-contaminated blood. The mucous membranes of the mouth and upper respiratory tract contribute to defense by trapping microorganisms within their sticky mucus. This layer of mucus is not easily crossed by HIV, so infection via the mouth or respiratory tract is an extremely rare event.

The acidity of the stomach provides a substantial barrier to infection of the intestines, and the acidity of the vaginal tract is a resistant barrier to microbes. Thus, HIV deposited in the vagina during sexual intercourse will not survive easily due to the acid environment, and the virus will not normally penetrate the muscular wall of this organ. However, if a woman has wounds or abrasions on the vaginal wall, then penetration may occur. Furthermore, if she has a sexually transmitted disease such as syphilis, gonorrhea, or chlamydia, the erosion of the tissue may encourage viral penetration.

An important antiviral substance of the body is interferon. Produced by numerous body cells in response to viral invasion, interferon triggers the production of inhibitory substances that interfere with viral reproduction. Interferons are a nonspecific mechanism of body defense. Some researchers are optimistic about them as a possibility for treatment of

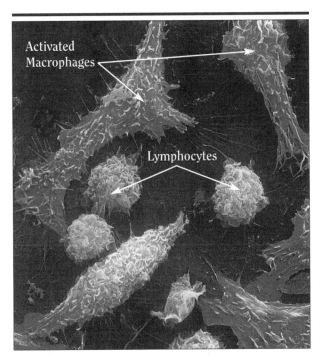

Activated
Macrophages

Lymphocytes

FIGURE 2.3 A scanning electron micrograph of some of the cells involved in the immune process. The activated macrophages set off the process, while the lymphocytes respond to the stimulation of the immune system.

viral diseases such as AIDS.

Within the body, there are numerous cells that engulf and destroy invading organisms by the process of phagocytosis. Among these cells are the neutrophils and monocytes of the circulatory system (Figure 2.3), and the macrophages of such tissues as the lymph nodes, spleen, brain, and bone marrow. Phagocytosis by these cells begins with the invagination and pinching-off of the cell membrane to form a bubblelike object called a phagocytic vesicle. The vesicle then fuses with an enzyme-laden lysosome within the cytoplasm, and digestive enzymes in the lysosome combine with the microorganism. The microorganism dissolves quickly, and the debris is left behind to be removed by cells of the reticuloendothelial system. Phagocytes operate against viruses, but sometimes the virus is able to infect the phagocyte and use it to make more viruses. Scientists have found that HIV fits this pattern of infection. As we shall see momentarily, phagocytosis is also an early step in the immune process.

Specific Resistance and the Immune System

As we previously noted, two major types of defense exist in the body to defend against microorganisms. The specific line of defense is centered in the body's immune system. Working with nonspecific mechanisms, the immune system is a key to eliminating pathogenic microorganisms from the body.

Four fundamental features underlie the immune system.

First, the immune response involves two sets of lymphocytes that act together with phagocytic cells. Second, the immune response is highly specific, meaning that a response to a disease confers resistance to that disease alone. Third, the immune response has memory, so once an immune response has been mounted to a microorganism, the second response to that organism is much more rapid and highly enhanced. Fourth, the immune response discriminates between the host (i.e., the human body) and the microbe that has stimulated it into action.

The chemical parts of the microbe that elicit an immune response are referred to as antigens. Most antigens are large molecules such as proteins and polysaccharides, and, on rare occasions, lipids or nucleic acids. Usually, antigenic substances are interpreted as being foreign to the body; in immunologic jargon, they are *nonself*. This concept implies that the immune system does not mount a response against substances it interprets as *self*. Essentially, everything that is not part of the body is considered nonself.

Although the immune response is directed to specific portions of the antigen molecule, known as antigenic determinants, we shall continue to refer to immune-stimulating agents in the larger context as "antigens." Antigens may include such things as bee venoms, bacterial toxins, the chemical components of HIV and other viruses, and virtually anything interpreted by the body as foreign. All antigens have two distinguishing properties: they stimulate immune system cells, and they react with the products of those cells or the cells themselves.

Activity of the Immune System

The immune system can mount a response to antigen through either or both of its two branches: antibody-mediated immunity (AMI) or cell-mediated immunity (CMI). Antibody-mediated immunity involves antibodies circulating in blood fluids such as blood, lymph, and mucous secretions at the body surfaces. Antibodies are produced through the intervention of B lymphocytes (also called B cells). Cell-mediated immunity is based on the activity of cells called sensitized T lymphocytes. T lymphocytes (also called T cells) act directly on foreign cells and destroy them. Cell-mediated immunity is most effective against the more complex eukaryotic microorganisms such as fungi and protozoa and against body cells infected by viruses and bacteria. By comparison, antibody-mediated immunity works against the less complex prokaryotic bacteria as well as viruses free in the body fluids.

As the major players in the immune system, B cells and T cells look very similar when viewed with the electron microscope. Both types of cells are lymphocytes—white blood cells with very large nuclei that encompass almost the entire cytoplasmic area. Lymphocytes make up about 30 percent of the cellular elements in the bloodstream, but the lymphocytes that function in the immune system are those in the lymph nodes, spleen, tonsils, and other lymphoid organs of the body.

Both B cells and T cells originate from stem cells in the bone marrow during the period of fetal development. T cells leave the bone marrow and pass through a lymphoid organ in the neck tissues known as the thymus. Here they are modified, and receptor sites composed of glycoprotein molecules are embedded at their surfaces. Different colonies of T cells emerge with different receptor sites. The sites react with the various antigens in the environment outside the body. After leaving the thymus, the T cells move through the circulation and colonize the lymph nodes of the neck, armpits, groin, and other parts of the body as well as the spleen and other lymphoid organs shown in Figure 2.4. These T cells are the target of infection by HIV.

B cells also emerge from the bone marrow at about the same time as the T cells. However, the B cells mature at a site believed to be the liver or bone marrow in humans. (In the embryonic chick, the maturation site is an organ along the gastrointestinal tract known as the bursa of Fabricius, hence the "B" for bursa.) During maturation, different colonies of B cells acquire different kinds of receptor sites for different types of antigens. These receptor sites represent the structure of the antibody that each B cell will produce. The B cells then move to the lymph nodes, spleen, and lymphoid organs, and colonize the organs together with the T cells. HIV particles will generally not attack B cells because the cells lack the receptor sites (the lock) that attract the virus (the key).

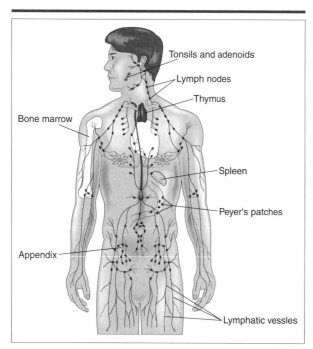

FIGURE 2.4 The names and locations of the major organs of the immune system. These organs contain the B cells and T cells that respond to stimulation by antigens. They are sites of infection by HIV.

When a virus or other microorganism enters the body, it is usually engulfed in phagocytosis by a white blood cell called the macrophage. The macrophage is a type of phagocytic cell in the tissues, as we have noted above. The phagocyte breaks down the microorganism into its component macromolecules and releases its antigens. The antigens are displayed on the macrophage surface as the macrophage circulates through the lymphatic and circulatory systems, eventually winding up in the lymph nodes or other lymphoid organ. The antigens are displayed within a set of proteins known as MHC proteins (for "major histocompatibility complex" proteins). The MHC proteins identify the macrophages as belonging to the human body and form a landscape for presenting the antigens to the cells of the immune system.

At the lymphoid tissues, the antigens stimulate either the B cells or T cells, depending upon the nature of the antigen and the presence of the correct receptor site on the cell. A type of T cell called the helper T cell is critical to the recognition. This cell serves as a type of gateway to the B and T cells. The helper T cell interacts with the antigen-bearing macrophage and "helps" the reaction take place between the macrophage and the responding T cell or B cell. Indeed, without the activity of the helper T cell, the overall immune response is severely depressed. Researchers have found that a primary target of HIV is the helper T cell, a finding that largely explains how HIV depresses the immune response.

At this point, the immune system diverges depending upon whether the B cells or T cells are stimulated. The results will be cell-mediated immunity (if T cells are stimulated) or antibody-mediated immunity (if B cells). Both types are displayed in Figure 2.5. When the T cells are stimulated into action, they become sensitized cells called cytotoxic T cells. These cells leave the lymphoid tissue and enter the lymph and blood. In a sense, the sensitized cells have a "picture" of the antigen they need to seek out and with which they will react. They travel to the infection site, where they encounter the fungus, protozoan, or other microorganisms. The cells interact directly with the microorganisms and exert a "lethal hit" on the microorganisms. They secrete enzymes that dissolve portions of the plasma membrane and cause the microorganism to leak its contents. They also secrete a number of active substances called cytokines (also called chemokines) that activate macrophages to engage in phagocytosis. The overall effect is to bring about a destruction of the virus or other antigen-bearing cells. As we shall see, when the T cells have been destroyed by HIV, the response to fungi, protozoa, and other microbes diminishes to the point of nonexistence.

In the lymphoid tissues, other antigens stimulate the B cells. Once stimulated, the B cells secrete protein molecules called antibodies. The B cells also mature into highly-active large cells called plasma cells, which continue the production of enormous numbers of antibody molecules (an estimated 2000 molecules of antibody per second).

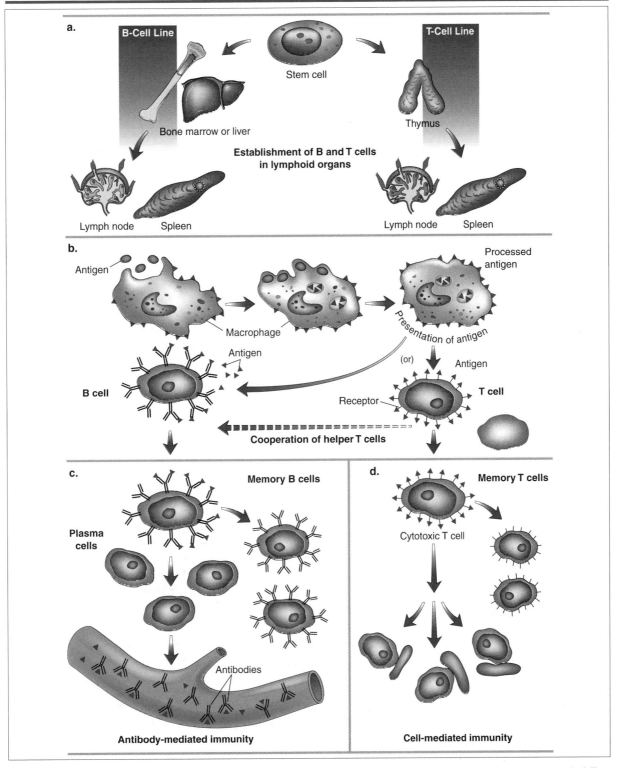

FIGURE 2.5 An overview of the immune system and its function. (a) Stem cells give rise to B cells and T cells through different pathways. Both cell types colonize the lymphoid organs. (b) Antigens from microbes are phagocytized and processed by
macrophages for presentation to B cells or T cells. (c) When B cells are stimulated, they revert to plasma cells, which produce antibody molecules released into the circulation for transport to the infection site. The result is antibody-mediated
immunity. (d) When T cells are stimulated, they revert to cytotoxic T cells that move to the infection site and interact with
microbes. The result is cell-mediated immunity. Memory B and T cells also form for later use should the microbes reenter
the body.

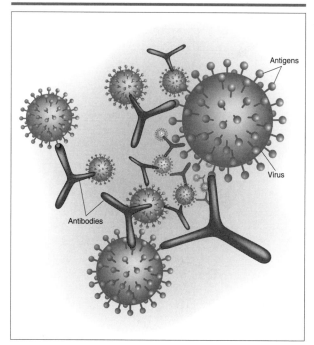

FIGURE 2.6 How antibodies work. Antibodies are protein molecules roughly shaped like the letter Y. At one end of the molecule, the antibody unites with the antigen on the surface of the microbe that had set off the immune process. When this happens on the viral surface, the virus cannot penetrate its host cell and replicate. Also the viral clump becomes an easy target for phagocytes. Unfortunately, HIV sequesters itself within host T cells, and antibodies cannot enter these cells.

Antibody molecules enter the bloodstream and fill the body fluids. At the infection site, they bind to the surfaces of viruses, much like strands of glue, and encourage clumping of the particles, as pictured in Figure 2.6. They also bind to the motion-associated flagella of bacteria and prevent the movement of these microbes, while also discouraging the microbe's adherence to the tissues. Furthermore, antibodies encourage phagocytosis by attaching viruses and bacteria to phagocytes. They also set off the complement cascade, a series of reactions involving multiple blood components that form compounds to drive molecular wedges into microbes, causing leakage to occur.

Antibodies are produced when a person has HIV infection, but the antibodies are unable to rid the body of the viruses, in part because the HIV penetrates T cells and antibody molecules do not enter these cells. These antibodies are those detected during the AIDS antibody test used for diagnostic purposes, as discussed in a later chapter. In many cases, such as during common cold infections, the antibody molecules are a key element in recovery. Sadly, the process does not work well in AIDS.

Once the antibodies have performed their immune function, the immune response will remain intact. Certain B cells become memory cells, remaining in the lymphoid tissues and beginning active secretion of antibodies should the antigens occur once again in the tissues. For this reason, few or no symptoms are experienced when microorganisms reenter the body. The body has become *immune*, a term meaning "free from."

Types of Immunity

The antibody response is also the basis for four different kinds of immunity that may exist in the body. These four types of immunity are known as acquired immunities because they develop after birth and are not part of nonspecific resistance. They include active natural immunity, active artificial immunity, passive natural immunity, and passive artificial immunity.

Active immunity comes about when the body produces its own antibodies. The active immunity is natural if the antibodies are produced in response to an infection, or it is artificial if the antibodies are produced in response to a vaccine. A vaccine contains inactivated viruses, weakened viruses, dead bacteria, or their parts. In all cases, the vaccine stimulates the immune system to produce antibodies that circulate in the body and provide a sentinel against the invasion by pathogenic microorganisms.

Immunity is regarded as passive immunity if antibodies are introduced to the person's bloodstream from an outside source. Passive immunity is natural when antibodies pass from mother to child during fetal development. The passive immunity is artificial if a person is given an injection of antibodies from the bloodstream of another individual.

As we have seen, the immune system plays the major role in specific body defense. Generations of medical researchers have known about the existence of the immune system, but its mechanisms of action remained somewhat obscure until the AIDS epidemic began in earnest. Then it became painfully clear to researchers and lay people that a body with a poorly functioning immune system is in trouble, deep trouble. The importance of the immune system will be even more clear in the chapters ahead.

Questions

1. Describe four considerations that are important in the establishment of infectious disease.

2. Summarize several of the mechanisms that lend non-specific resistance in the human body.

3. Explain the role of the immune system in specific resistance and outline the process by which each of its two branches operates.

Chapter Three

The Biology of HIV

Review and Preview

We now have sufficient information to discuss viruses in general and the human immunodeficiency virus (HIV) as it relates to AIDS. Part of the foundation was set in Chapter 1, where we discussed how AIDS emerged and when it was first observed. In the early years, HIV remained unidentified, but health professionals recognized that something unusual and serious was taking place. After HIV was discovered by a French group of investigators, attention focused on prevention and treatment. Unfortunately, AIDS continued to spread even as researchers hunted for new drugs and medicines, and by the late 1990s, about 30 million people worldwide were living with HIV infection and/or AIDS.

As noted in Chapter 1, research evidence indicates that HIV probably originated in a subspecies of chimpanzee and that it had entered human populations as early as 1959, probably by direct contact with a chimpanzee. As the disease continued to spread, biologists such as Paul Ewald pointed out that behavioral and social changes in the 1960s probably encouraged spread of the virus and that behavioral and social changes could halt its spread.

Chapter 2 placed AIDS in the context of infectious disease and the immune system. We saw that HIV, like other viruses, enters the body by a specific mode, has a certain dose level required for establishment of disease, fits into a molecular lock on its host T cell, then follows a pattern of infection found in with many other diseases. The immune system is the essential feature in specific body defense, and it involves two branches, one centered in antibodies and the other involving cytotoxic T cells. As major players in the immune system, the B cells and T cells are responsible for the production of antibodies and cytotoxic T cells, respectively, and the helper T cells are a key to activating the system of immunity. As we shall see in this chapter, the helper T cells are vulnerable to infection by HIV. As their numbers decline, HIV infection progresses to acquired immune deficiency syndrome, or AIDS.

In this chapter, we shall also examine some details of HIV. The virus has a shape and size within the framework of other viruses; its symmetry is described as icosahedral. HIV, like other viruses, replicates only within living cells. In the case of HIV, the living cell is often the helper T cell, also called the CD4+ cell. We shall discuss the general process of replication and show that the T cells can be rapidly destroyed when HIV is present. Some specific characteristics make HIV unique, such as its genes. We shall also talk about the receptors by which HIV recognizes its host T cell. This recognition is a critical feature in viral replication, and it is intensely studied by researchers, because if the recognition can be prevented, then replication can be interrupted.

The chapter will conclude with an acknowledgment of how difficult it is to study viruses, as they must be cultivated in living tissue. This cultivation is considerably different than for bacteria, where artificial laboratory gels can be used. The difficulty in cultivating viruses makes working with HIV particularly burdensome.

Introduction

Viruses are among the smallest microbes capable of infecting a host and replicating in the host's cells. The tiniest viruses, such as the polioviruses, are an incredibly small 20 nanometers in diameter (a nanometer is a billionth of a meter). The largest viruses approximate the smallest bacteria in size and are barely visible with the bright-field microscope. They are typified by poxviruses, which are about 250 nanometers in diameter. In between these extremes, there exist many different types of viruses and an equally large variety in sizes. The human immunodeficiency virus (HIV) is among the smaller viruses known to science. The pages ahead examine its biology.

 ## The Structure of Viruses and HIV

All viruses are composed of one or more molecules of nucleic acid tightly encased in a protein coat and in some viruses, a membranelike envelope. The coat (and envelope, when present) protect the nucleic acid and help the virus bind to its host cell. HIV is an example of an enveloped virus.

The nucleic acid component of the virus is known as its genome, a term that refers to the total of all genes. The viral genome can be composed of ribonucleic acid (RNA) or deoxyribonucleic acid (DNA), but it never contains both. The nucleic acid may occur as a double-stranded molecule (i.e., a double helix), or it may be single-stranded, as in the HIV. A virus is often referred to as a "DNA virus" or an "RNA virus" according to the nucleic acid content of its genome. HIV is an example of an RNA virus, having two molecules of the nucleic acid in its genome.

In some viruses such as HIV, the genome is organized as a linear nucleic acid molecule, whereas in others the molecule is a closed loop. The genome may contain several hundred genes as in the larger viruses or fewer than 10, as found in HIV. There is no cytoplasm in a virus, nor are there any organelles, granules, or other structures found in microbial and more complex eukaryotic cells (such as human cells). However, some viruses have enzyme molecules associated with their genome. HIV is an example: it contains two molecules of an enzyme called reverse transcriptase that mingle among the RNA molecules of its genome. During the replication cycle, this enzyme catalyzes the formation of a DNA molecule, using the RNA molecule as a template (model). We shall discuss this process presently.

The protein coat enclosing the viral genome is called the capsid, and the combination of genome and capsid is termed the nucleocapsid as Figure 3.1 shows. Capsids are constructed from a large number of protein subunits called capsomeres. Hundreds of capsomeres exist in the capsid but there are very few different kinds, a reflection of the few genes present in the genome. Capsomeres are stitched together to form the capsid much as the patches form a quilt.

The geometric configuration of the capsid can be a helix or a polyhedron. When the capsid follows the helical symmetry of the nucleic acid, the capsid takes the shape of a helix. Tobacco mosaic viruses, the agents of mosaic disease in tobacco plants, are an example of viruses with helical symmetry. The polyhedron is a multifaceted geometric shape. For many viruses, it is a 20-sided figure called an icosahedron. Each side of the icosahedron is a triangular face composed of capsomeres. Viruses such as herpesviruses, polioviruses, and mononucleosis viruses have icosahedral symmetry.

When it is first produced, HIV has an icosahedral shape, but the shape of the virus converts rapidly to that of a cone. In 1998, researchers from the University of Utah presented data on how the core of HIV is formulated. They presented high-resolution electron micrographs of cross-sections showing a hollow tube composed of pure capsid. The micrographs indicate that the tube walls are a honeycomb of hexagonal rings consisting of capsid molecules, or capsomeres. The

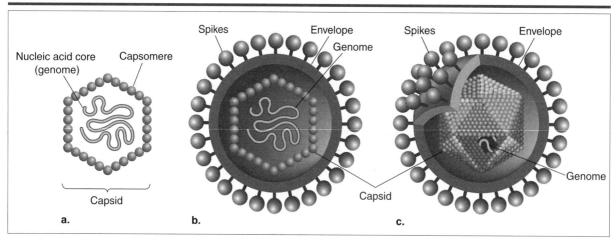

FIGURE 3.1   Construction of an icosahedral virus. (a) The nucleic acid core (the genome) surrounded by a capsid composed of capsomeres. (b) The nucleocapsid (genome plus capsid) enclosed by an envelope with spikes. (c) A three-dimensional view of an isoahedral virus.

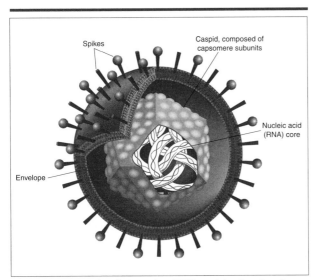

FIGURE 3.2 A stylized view of an HIV particle showing its icosahedral symmetry and envelope with spikes.

researchers suggested that the addition of capsomere molecules together with RNA could tilt the rows of hexagons into a spiral. This would force the entire structure to become narrow toward one end and form the conelike core of the virus. Figure 3.2 illustrates HIV before this reversion occurs.

The membranous covering associated with many viruses is the envelope. It is found in such viruses as herpesviruses, influenza viruses, and HIV. The envelope is derived from the membrane of the host cell at the conclusion of the replication cycle, but it is not identical to the host membrane because it contains viral-specified proteins.

In addition, some viruses such as HIV have projections of the envelope known as spikes. The spikes of HIV have been studied intensely because protein molecules in the spikes react with host cell membranes during host cell attachment. Two glycoproteins called glycoprotein 120 (gp120) and glycoprotein 41 (gp41) are both found in the envelope. These glycoproteins form a tight recognition with receptor sites on the surface of helper T cells, which form a basic underpinning of the immune system. We will discuss this interaction presently.

 ## Viral Physiology and Classification

Viruses are said to be obligate intracellular parasites. This description implies that viruses are "obliged" to replicate within ("intra") the host cell. Indeed, viruses cannot replicate apart from cells. Put another way, viruses are inert particles outside the confines of living cells. Researchers have a difficult time studying viruses because they are much more difficult to maintain in the lab than are bacteria, fungi, or protozoa. The latter groups can be cultivated on artificial laboratory media, but for viruses some type of cellular life must be employed as a culture medium.

In contrast to bacteria and other microbial groups, viruses have no widely accepted system of classification. Various committees of virologists have proposed numerous classification systems that use such characteristics as type of nucleic acid, size, capsid geometry, presence or absence of an envelope, nature of the host, and nature of the reproductive process. As yet, however, no one system is universally accepted. Instead, virologists often refer to viruses according to the type of tissue they infect. They recognize animal viruses, plant viruses, and bacterial viruses (viruses that replicate within bacteria). In this context, the HIV is considered an animal virus.

Despite the absence of a formal classification system, virologists have placed viruses into such families as Picornaviridae (small RNA viruses, including the poliovirus), Herpesviridae (large DNA viruses, including the herpes simplex virus), and Retroviridae (viruses that synthesize DNA using RNA as a template, including HIV).

Replication of Viruses and HIV

Viruses replicate only within a host cell. Apart from this cell, a virus is nothing more than a few genes packaged in protein. When the virus encounters its host cell, however, it is able to reproduce at a highly efficient rate.

Each virus type can infect only a limited type of host cells. This specificity during the attachment phase depends on the existence of recognition sites at the surface of host cell. Viruses identify these so-called "receptor sites," and a match is made during the recognition phase. During HIV infection, the gp120 and gp41 molecules of the HIV envelope recognize a receptor site called the CD4 site on the cell membrane of cells, such as an immune system component known as a helper T cell (or helper T lymphocyte). The gp120, gp41, and CD4 proteins promote the fusion of the viral envelope and the plasma membrane of the helper T cell into a continuous layer of membrane. This action permits the viral core to enter the cytoplasm of the cell. (Other surface molecules, or coreceptors, are also involved, as we will see presently.) In the medical literature the helper T cell is called a "CD4+ cell" because of the presence of the receptor.

The viral genome enters the cytoplasm of the cell during the penetration phase. The fusion of the viral envelope with the cell membrane is followed by the opening of a passageway into the cytoplasm. In viruses without an envelope, the cell brings the virus into its cytoplasm via phagocytosis.

Once the virus is within the cytoplasm of the host cell, enzymes in the host cell dissolve the protein capsid and release the viral genome. Entry of the genome into the host's cytoplasm constitutes the infection phase. Now, either of two processes may occur. In some cases, the genome encodes viral proteins, and new viruses are rapidly produced in the host cell. Huge numbers of viruses are quickly produced, and the cell is often destroyed in this process. The symptoms of disease can arise from the cellular death and destruction. This cycle is referred to as the lytic (lit'ik) cycle of reproduction because it results in death to the host cell by lysis (meaning "breaking open").

The second pattern of the infection phase is called the lysogenic (ly-so-gen'ik) cycle. It occurs in HIV and several other viruses such as herpesviruses. In this process, the virus does not reproduce immediately. Instead, the virus uses its enzyme reverse transcriptase to synthesize a molecule of DNA, using the RNA as a template (Figure 3.3). The newly-formed DNA sequence has nitrogenous bases (e.g., A,G,C,T) complementing those in the viral RNA. The DNA produced in this manner is called a provirus. Because this chemistry is a reversal of the normal RNA production from the DNA code, the virus is called a retrovirus, and the enzyme is termed reverse transcriptase.

Once the provirus has been produced, it moves to the cell nucleus and integrates into the DNA found here. As part of the chromosomal material, the provirus then replicates when the cell undergoes mitosis (reproduction), and copies pass to new cells. The person so infected with HIV is said to have "HIV infection." HIV integration into the DNA of a host T cell appears to be a random process. It can occur anywhere within open fragments of chromosomal material. Research evidence indicates that HIV can infect a cell only when the cell is actively dividing. The viruses may survive for a period of time in a cell, but it cannot insert its proviral DNA into the cell's DNA unless the cell is undergoing division. This may be the reason why some individuals at high risk of contracting HIV do not become infected; that is, they may have escaped infection because the virus cannot insert its DNA into cells that are not dividing.

Public health officials have estimated that approximately 1 million Americans carry HIV in its DNA form (the provirus) and have HIV infection. Because blood, semen, vaginal fluid, and breast milk carry T cells, the disease can be transmitted at this stage by infected T cells.

There are many variations of the lytic and lysogenic cycle occurring in animal, plant, and bacterial cells, but the common thread is that viruses utilize the biochemical machinery of the cell for their own purposes. Genes in the provirus encode enzymes that use cellular amino acids for proteins. These proteins may be used to synthesize new viral capsids and nucleic acids for constructing viral genomes. The viruses use the cell's ribosomes (submicroscopic particles of RNA) for the construction of new proteins; they employ the cell's membranes for storing the proteins; and they appropriate its cellular enzymes for modifying the proteins. In general terms, the viruses divert the host cell resources for their own purposes in an ultimate act of parasitism.

After viral genomes and capsomeres have been synthesized, the assembly phase begins. In the assembly phase, the capsid proteins are trimmed to the proper size by the enzyme protease. (This enzyme is the site of action by the new protease inhibitor drugs.) Next the genomes and capsids are brought together to form new viral particles. Viruses such as HIV then modify the cell's membrane with viral proteins, move to the cell surface, and emerge from the cell by forcing their way through the membrane. This process, called budding, is where HIV obtains its envelope as Figure 3.4 displays. In some cases, the host cell disintegrates as it releases the viruses, because the holes can result in cytoplasmic leakage and death. However, the host cell may remain alive if it can repair its membrane damage quickly.

The HIV Genome

As noted above, the genome is the total number of all the genes possessed by an entity such as a virus. There are at least nine recognizable genes in the HIV genome, including three that researchers have studied in depth. The first gene is *gag* (short for "*g*roup-specific *a*nti*g*en"), which encodes a protein cleaved by the enzyme protease into four separate proteins for use in viral capsid construction. The second is *pol* (short for *pol*ymerase). This gene encodes at least three enzymes including viral protease, reverse transcriptase, and integrase, the enzyme used for inserting the provirus into the host genome.

The third gene is *env* (short for *env*elope). This gene encodes a 160 kilodalton protein later cleaved by a protease enzyme to produce the two glycoproteins mentioned above.

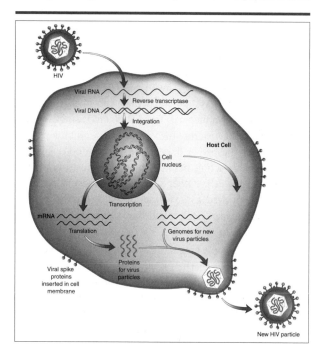

FIGURE 3.3 How HIV replicates. The viral RNA is set free in the host cell cytoplasm, and reverse transcriptase synthesizes a complementary molecule of DNA. The latter integrates to the cell nucleus, from which it programs the synthesis of proteins and genomes for new viral particles via translation using mRNA. The nucleocapsids bud through the cell membrane and acquire their envelopes.

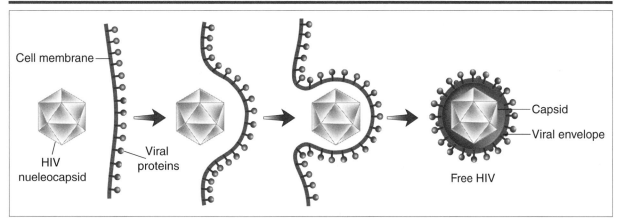

FIGURE 3.4 How HIV acquires its envelope. Near the end of the replication process, the HIV nucleocapsid moves to the cell membrane where viral proteins have been inserted. The nucleocapsid forces its way through the membrane and encloses itself in the viral-marked membrane.

The first glycoprotein, gp120, extends out from the viral envelope and contacts a receptor on the host T cell where the virus attaches. This receptor, the CD4 protein, exists not only on helper T cells but also on white blood cells called monocytes. Monocytes are the precursors of macrophages, the phagocytic cells used in the immune process (Chapter 2). The second protein, gp41, remains within the viral envelope as a transmembrane protein and anchors the gp120 molecule to the envelope of the virus.

In addition to these three genes, the genome includes long-terminal-repeat (LTR) sequences at both ends of the genome. LTRs are repeating sequences of bases in the nucleic acid. Also, the genome contains the regulatory and auxiliary genes *tat, rev, nef, vif, vpu,* and *vpr.* The *tat* gene appears to regulate the expression of viral mRNA. When the *tat* protein is present, additional mRNA is transcribed during the protein synthesis process, and additional HIV RNA is produced. The second gene, *rev,* appears to enhance the stability of the three main genes in the genome.

Scientists have found that the gene *nef* apparently shields HIV from the human immune system and allows the infection to progress toward AIDS. The gene seems to reduce or erase the surface proteins used as distress signals when a cell is infected. These surface proteins are the antigens that interact with immune system cells. This cell displays these antigens when it is infected. This process was discovered through studies of AIDS patients in Australia. These individuals, who had been infected by a blood transfusion, had apparently contracted a version of HIV lacking *nef.* Accordingly, they did not progress to AIDS, even after years of infection. This study suggests that *nef* has a role to play in controlling the virulence of HIV. The *nef* gene may thus decrease the level of viral mRNA and act as a regulatory protein. This action reduces the virulence of HIV. From an evolutionary standpoint, the gene is valuable because it helps keep the host cell alive for a longer period of time so that the virus can produce more offspring.

The gene *vif* is an infectivity factor that helps spread the virus between cells. The gene encodes proteins that increase the infectiousness of the virus after it has budded from the host T cell. Viruses sometimes spread from cell to cell by fusion of the two cells, and the protein encoded by *vif* may assist the virus when it is released outside its host T cell. The *vpu* and *vpr* genes also work within the replication cycle.

Although the viral genome is generally stable, changes may develop as a result of errors made by the enzyme reverse transcriptase. This occurs during the synthesis of DNA using the viral RNA as a model (template). The mutations encourage the virus to exist in many different combinations of proteins and genes. Evolutionary forces through natural selection choose the fittest virus from among the available mutants, and this selection may account for HIV's emergence as a human pathogen. The effects of the mutations are important considerations in the development of drugs and therapies to counteract HIV.

HIV and Cell Receptors

In 1986, Paul Maddon of Columbia University identified the CD4 surface protein as the receptor for HIV and the point used by HIV for entering cells. (The title CD4 stands for "cluster designation number 4.") However, in subsequent years, scientists studying the interaction between HIV and its host T cell found evidence that CD4 is not the only important factor for HIV entry. When mouse cells were genetically engineered to produce human CD4 molecules, HIV could bind to the cells but not enter them.

In recent years, scientists have learned that at least one additional surface antigen receptor is required for entry of HIV into cells. The CD26 receptor site was discovered in 1993 by French researchers led by Ara Hovanessian at the Pasteur Institute in Paris. In laboratory mice that do not naturally produce CD4 and/or CD26, researchers discovered that the mouse cells became vulnerable to HIV once they were genetically engineered to produce both CD4 and CD26. When either receptor was absent, HIV infection failed to occur.

Further research has elucidated how CD26 apparently functions together with CD4. The CD26 receptor is an enzyme having a signal peptide (a small protein) acting as a membrane-anchoring domain. Research evidence indicates that as HIV approaches the T cell, the gp120 molecule binds to the CD4 receptor molecule. This action exposes an amino acid chain in the gp120 complex called the V3 loop. The loop now extends out from the gp120 complex and interacts with the CD26 receptor. Acting as a peptidase enzyme, the receptor splits the amino acid chain in the V3 loop, and the reaction results in biochemical changes that permit the gp41 molecule to interact with the cellular membrane. Cell and virus fusion follows quickly, and the nucleocapsid of the HIV particle enters the cell's cytoplasm.

However, the place of CD26 in AIDS pathology is not universally accepted. When the data were published, many scientists pointed out flaws in the research and thus viewed the results with skepticism. As of this time, it is not clear whether CD26 is a coreceptor for HIV, although many scientists continue to work on that possibility.

Another discovery made in 1996 shed additional light on the interaction between HIV and its host T cell. Researchers at the National Institutes of Health (NIH) identified a previously unknown coreceptor, a cell surface molecule on the T cell that they named "fusin" (because it permits cells to fuse with the surface of HIV). By that time, it was well-known that HIV attacks a human cell by attaching its envelope protein (gp120) to the CD4 molecule. But, the researchers discovered, infection does not occur unless the virus also connects with the fusin molecule. That is, HIV cannot invade cells by means of the CD4 receptor alone, but it readily infects cells having CD4 and fusin. Entry, they maintained, is a multistage interplay between HIV and two receptors found on the surface of the T cell: the CD4 receptor and fusin receptor. After first binding to the CD4 receptor, the virus attaches to the second receptor, fusin.

Edward Berger of the NIH continued the research and that same year, he reported that fusin is identical to the molecule known as CXCR4. Subsequent studies have shown that CXCR4 (fusin) is one of several chemokine receptors (discussed below), which are used by different strains of HIV to infect T cells. Scientists now speculate that, after the CD4 receptor and gp120 molecule bind to one another, the complex undergoes a structural change to twist and expose different parts of the complex. The complex then binds to the coreceptor CXCR4 (fusin). After the CXCR4 (fusin) binds to the CD4–gp120 complex, the bottom part of gp41 is released to attach to the cell membrane. The CXCR4 (fusin) thus chaperones the HIV nucleocapsid into the cell by allowing the gp41 molecule to breach the cell membrane. Figure 3.5 illustrates the process.

HIV and Chemokine Receptors

In the late 1980s, virologists first reported that certain T cells can prevent the replication of HIV. These cells are known as CD8 cells. They are often referred to as suppressor T cells. Researchers postulated that the cells interfere with HIV replication by secreting an unidentified factor or factors. Then, in 1995, Robert Gallo and his colleagues reported that three closely related polypeptides work together to inhibit HIV. The polypeptides are a group of lymphocyte-produced proteins called chemokines (also called lymphokines and cytokines). In laboratory cultures, the chemokines were able to inhibit the replication of HIV.

In the 1980s, researcher Jay Levy had found that the level of chemokines declines as HIV-infected patients progress to AIDS. In his 1995 work, Gallo and his fellow researchers showed that pure versions of the compounds could suppress viral replication when added to HIV-infected T cells. They also showed that the suppressor effect was eliminated by the action of highly specific antibodies produced against the chemokines.

Later, in 1996 a group of scientists reported that the HIV strain most commonly found in humans infects cells by using a signal protein on the surface of T cells that they called CC-CKR-5. They soon discovered that CC-CKR-5 binds to chemokines, the three proteins secreted by CD8 cells (and studied by Gallo).

The research was further stimulated by the observation that some individuals are frequently exposed to HIV but remain HIV-negative, possibly because they secrete high amounts of the three chemokines. Similar results were obtained from a study of hemophiliac individuals who remained uninfected despite having received HIV-contaminated blood. The chemokines may physically block the access of HIV to the CC-CKR-5 protein site. Alternately, the chemokines may signal a cell to remove such proteins from its surface. Thus, CC-CKR-5 presents a tantalizing target for drugs to deny HIV access to cells.

Current scientific thinking is that the absence of CC-CKR-5 protein may determine that an individual is genetically immune to AIDS. In 1996, two high-risk men were studied for their apparent immunity to AIDS. Scientists reported that both men were missing the CC-CKR-5 protein, that the genes for encoding the protein were defective. Approximately 1 percent of Americans of Western European descent are believed to carry two copies of the defective gene on chromosome number 3. This defect apparently protects them against invasion by HIV. About 22 percent of the same ethnic category have one copy of the mutated gene. The defective CC-CKR-5 gene does not appear to have any other unusual effects on those who possess it.

The mutations of the CC-CKR-5 gene help explain some puzzling cases in which individuals exposed to HIV remained uninfected. The discovery also strengthens the hypothesis

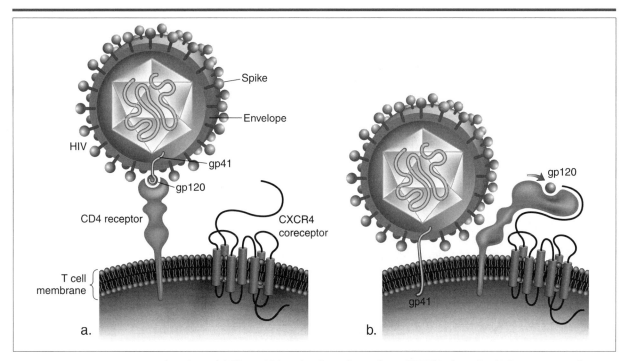

FIGURE 3.5 How a coreceptor functions. (a) The gp120 molecule at the surface of HIV binds to the CD4 receptor on the T cell surface. (b) Then the complex twists and shifts away to bind to the coreceptor CXCR4. This twisting exposes the gp41 molecule, which attaches to the T cell membrane. Entry of the HIV nucleocapsid follows.

that drugs interfering with the reaction between HIV and CC-CKR-5 can slow the spread of virus in infected individuals. The mutation in the CC-CKR-5 gene consist of a large gap in the DNA of the gene. The gap leads to a shortened or incomplete protein that the virus cannot use. Investigators speculate that resistant individuals inherit one mutant copy of the gene from each parent. Apparently the mutation is common in some human populations but rare in others, which suggests a rather recent evolutionary origin of the mutation. However, scientists caution that several HIV strains use molecules other than CC-CKR-5 to infect T cells.

In addition to its role in virus-cell fusion, the CC-CKR-5 protein is a reaction site for the three immune-signaling chemokines that suppress HIV infection. Chemokines are involved in the body's inflammatory response. They may suppress HIV infectivity by blocking the fusion used by the virus to enter cells. This discovery has raised hopes for developing new AIDS therapies or vaccines. For example, it might be possible to prevent HIV from infecting cells by mimicking the way chemokines suppress HIV infectivity by blocking the site that they and HIV share.

Types of HIV

Throughout the world, most AIDS patients are infected with HIV-1. Over the years it has become clear that a second virus, HIV-2, is responsible for a mild form of AIDS that occurs primarily in West Africa, as noted in Chapter 1.

HIV-1 is further subdivided into two genetically distinct groups. The first group is designated group *M* for "major" group. The second group is designated group *O* for "outlier" group. The M group accounts for the overwhelming majority of infection with HIV-1. The O group is found almost exclusively in Cameroon, Africa. Each of these groups is then split into various subtypes according to geographical distribution and RNA sequence.

In 1998, researchers in France reported a new variant, which appeared to be an entirely separate third group of HIV. The new strain is designated ybf30. When the sequence of bases in the genome of ybf30 was determined, the results confirmed that it belongs to a previously unknown group. The researchers have proposed calling the group the N group. Analysis of the genome places it closer on the evolutionary tree to SIV than to either M or O group of HIV-1.

The various types of HIV continue to exact a significant toll of sickness and death throughout the world. For example, the World Health Organization (WHO) reported that, in 1999, 2.6 million people worldwide died of AIDS and its related causes, and 33.6 million were living with HIV infection or AIDS (Figure 3.6). Indeed, of the latter number, 5.6 million people became infected in 1999 alone, the greatest majority in sub-Saharan Africa. For those who believe the global pandemic is on the wane, WHO reported that the number of people living with HIV/AIDS was an increase over 1998, when 33.4 million were afflicted.

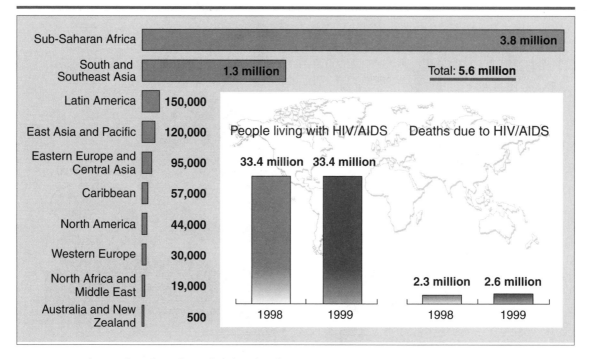

FIGURE 3.6   The number of people newly infected with HIV in 1999, as reported by the World Health Organization.

Viral Cultivation

Three types of cell cultures (or tissue cultures) are used in clinical research to maintain and propagate viruses. Primary cell cultures are one type. This culture consists of cells obtained directly from animal tissues. The cells support numerous types of viruses. Indeed, different viruses display a distinctive cytopathic effect (CPE) on the cells, a phenomenon useful for diagnostic purposes. Measles viruses, for example, cause the cells in a primary culture to form masses of giant cells called syncytia (sin-sish'a, plural of syncytium). This phenomenon also happens within the body.

A second type of cell culture is the diploid fibroblast culture. This culture consists of immature cells called fibroblasts. The cells are derived from fetal tissues and retain the capacity for rapid and repeated cell division, a property not present in primary cell cultures.

The third type of culture is the continuous cell line culture. The cells in this culture have been propagated for many generations and are less difficult to cultivate than normal cells because they have adapted to laboratory conditions. Note that in all instances, viruses multiply within the host cells of the culture. Technically, it is incorrect to refer to the process of "growing viruses" because viruses do not grow.

HIV's Affect on Cells

Within the retrovirus family, HIV is classified as a lentivirus with genetic and morphologic similarities to animal lentiviruses such as those that infect cats, sheep, goats, and primates. These animal viruses primarily infect cells of the immune system, including T cells and macrophages. Lentiviruses often cause immunodeficiency in their hosts in addition to slow, progressive wasting disorders with neurodegeneration and death. In Macaque (ma-kak') monkeys HIV causes wasting, diarrhea, opportunistic illnesses, T cell depletion, and death.

Several mechanisms of T cell killing have been observed in the laboratory for lentiviruses, and they may explain the progressive loss of cells in HIV-infected individuals. These mechanisms include disruption of the cell membrane as HIV buds from the surface of the cell (Figure 3.7), or the intracellular accumulation of RNA and DNA molecules associated with viral replication. The complexing of products from CD4+ cells and viral envelopes can also result in cell killing. Of course, the direct HIV-mediated cytopathic effect is responsible for most single cell killing.

The formation of syncytia contributes to cell death. A syncytium (sin-sish'ee-um) is the result of the binding together of infected cells to yield a functionless cell mass. During syncytium formation, uninfected cells infuse with infected cells, resulting in giant cells. Also, uninfected cells may be killed when free gp120 molecules from the envelope protein bind to the surface of the cells and mark them for destruction by cytotoxic T cells, as Chapter 2 explains.

The untimely induction of a form of programmed cell death called apoptosis (a-po-to'sis) has been proposed as an additional mechanism for T cell loss. The role of apoptosis in the development of the embryo has been known for decades,

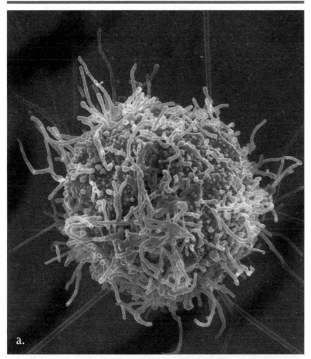

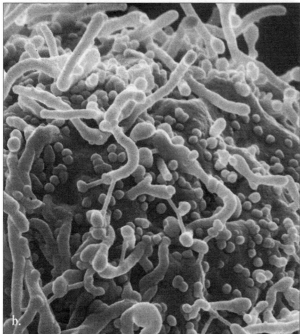

FIGURE 3.7   HIV and its host cell. **(a)** A scanning electron micrograph of a human T cell with infecting viral particles at its surface (magnification, ×7000). **(b)** A closeup view showing numerous viral particles budding from the surface (magnification, ×20,000).

but the importance of apoptosis in the daily maintenance of organisms has only been studied since the early 1970s. In 1972, Australian pathologists first proposed that the same type of cell death going on during embryonic development also happens in mature organisms and continues throughout life. They suggested that programmed cell death is an active process requiring energy expenditure, and that inhibition of apoptosis could contribute to several diseases. For example, it is widely believed today that failure of apoptosis encourages cancer.

Induction of apoptosis in healthy cells is believed to contribute to the immune deficiency associated with AIDS. It is known, for instance, that helper T cells and cytotoxic T cells die in an individual infected with HIV. Scientists now recognize that many more T cells die than are infected with HIV. It is possible that the cell's inability to make protein after viral infection may induce apoptosis, a form of cell suicide. Evolutionarily speaking, if the whole cell dies, the virus is eliminated. Thus, certain viruses have developed ways to inhibit apoptosis. The Epstein-Barr virus, which is involved in infectious mononucleosis, is believed to encode a protein to inhibit apoptosis.

One theory suggests that the suicide of T cells may arise from the release of gp120 proteins from HIV. Research evidence indicates that the gp120 protein attaches to CD4 molecules on the surface of T cells, and that the bound gp120–CD4 complex attracts HIV antibodies. The union with antibodies may prime a cell to kill itself. This theory is in its early stage, but it remains enticing possibility to explain the death of cells after HIV infection. This cell death is the ultimate cause of the symptoms of HIV infection and AIDS, as we explore in Chapter 4.

Questions

1. Summarize the structure of the human immunodeficiency virus (HIV) with emphasis on its three main parts and their chemical makeup.

2. Describe in detail the process by which HIV replicates in a host T cell.

3. Discuss the importance of cell receptors and chemokines in the replication of HIV and indicate the current thinking on these issues in the scientific community.

Chapter Four

How HIV Affects the Body

Review and Preview

With the 1984 identification of human immunodeficiency virus (HIV), public health entered a new phase in which acquired immune deficiency syndrome (AIDS) was first characterized as an infectious disease. Scientists could now use laboratory studies of the virus to help determine its action in the body, while they continued their work on effective treatments, cures, and vaccines. As the years passed, however, it became apparent that AIDS was not a short-range problem, but rather an epidemic—indeed, a pandemic—that would continue for many decades to come. The millions of individuals infected throughout the world, as well as the mounting death toll has ensured that AIDS will remain prominent in the public consciousness well into the 21st century.

Through their studies, researchers have found that HIV probably originated from a subspecies of the chimpanzee, and that many strains of HIV now exist. The spread of these strains could probably be related to the behavioral and social changes that began to occur during the 1960s and continued through to the present day.

AIDS fits the general pattern of an infectious disease, and many factors that attend other diseases are associated with AIDS. The primary focus of HIV is on the specific resistance mechanisms of the body, notably the immune system. The branch of the system supported by the B cells is only mildly affected, but the branch founded on T cells is profoundly altered. The body uses helper T cells as a gateway to both antibody-mediated and cell-mediated immunity, and it produces cytotoxic T cells to ward off infections by protozoa, fungi, virus-infected cells, cancer cells, and other such cells. The cytotoxic T cells attack microorganisms directly and secrete a number of substances called cytokines that activate macrophages and encourage them to perform phagocytosis, while calling other body defenses into action. The overall effect is to bring about an end to the infection.

The human immunodeficiency virus (HIV) begins with an icosahedral symmetry, then matures to the shape of a cone. Its core consists of two RNA molecules and two molecules of reverse transcriptase, surrounded by a protein capsid, which is divided into protein subunits called capsomeres. Surrounding the capsid is an envelope containing spikes with two glycoproteins. During its replication cycle, HIV associates with the CD4 receptor site and other sites on the surface of the helper T cell, and the nucleocapsid enters the cell cytoplasm. At this point, reverse transcriptase encodes DNA, using the RNA genome as a template. The viral DNA integrates to the DNA of the cell nucleus as a provirus, and the infected individual develops a condition called HIV infection. From the site, the provirus encodes the proteins needed for the replication of HIV. As the new nucleocapsids force their way through the cell membrane, they acquire their envelopes.

Scientists have now identified certain critical genes of HIV including three genes entitled *env, pol,* and *gag.* In the previous chapter, we discussed the key proteins encoded by these genes as well as several others whose synthesis is directed by the HIV genome. We finished with a discussion of some of the various ways that HIV affects its host T cell. These include formation of a syncytium, as well as budding and the general deterioration of a cell resulting from viral replication. In this chapter we will examine some of the profound effects this T cell destruction has on the body.

As this reading progresses, note that early in the infection the viruses are continually being produced, but the body is able to keep up with their numbers and destroy them. Eventually however, HIV overwhelms the body and the destruction of T cells becomes too substantial to sustain a defense to disease. At that time, opportunistic illnesses ensue, and the infected individual progresses to AIDS. Other illnesses associated with AIDS, including dementia and the wasting syndrome, will also be discussed as we develop an image of how infection with HIV brings on AIDS.

Introduction

As early as 1981, scientists realized that HIV has its primary affects on the body's immune system. An important clue was the observation that infection with HIV causes patients to develop diseases related to an impaired immune system. For example, patients were developing a form of pneumonia caused by an opportunistic organism called *Pneumocystis carinii* (new"mo-sis'tis car-in'e-e). This disease is normally quite rare in humans, but it occurs in patients whose immune system has been damaged.

Another clue that AIDS involves the immune system was found by examining tissue samples of AIDS patients. The damage to immune tissue was substantial, and scientists realized that they were seeing a pathologic condition rarely seen elsewhere. (At the time, HIV had not yet been identified or cultivated.) Organs of the immune system are located throughout the body and are generally referred to as lymphoid organs. This nomenclature is based on the role of the lymphoid organs in the development and function of lymphocytes, a type of white blood cell. The lymphoid organs include the bone marrow, thymus, lymph nodes, spleen, tonsils, and adenoids. Lymphatic vessels that transport lymphocytes to other structures of the body are also considered part of the lymphatic system.

Organs of the immune system are the primary focus of HIV. With the gradual deterioration of these organs and their cells, the symptoms of HIV infection develop, then AIDS follows. We will discuss this progression in the pages ahead.

Cell Pathologies

As discussed in Chapter 2, the lymphoid organs contain two types of immune cells: the T cells (technically, T lymphocytes) and the B cells (technically, B lymphocytes). B cells respond to antigens derived from bacteria, viruses, and other chemicals in the environment; on stimulation, they mature to plasma cells, which produce complex proteins called antibodies. T cells respond somewhat differently; on stimulation, certain T cells mature to cytotoxic T cells that enter the circulation and respond to antigens from fungi, protozoa, transplanted cells, tumor cells, and cells that carry foreign substances within them (such as virus-infected cells). The T cells interact cell to cell, and they kill the cell that contains the antigens.

But before all this happens another type of T cell is called into action. A key class of T cells are the helper T cells, which regulate the development of both B cells and cytotoxic T cells. The helper T cell is also referred to as a "CD4+ cell" because it contains on its surface a molecule called the CD4 receptor site, as well as other coreceptors discussed in Chapter 3. The helper T cell is so-named because it "helps" the B cell when it recognizes antigens as they come into the lymphoid organs. HIV replicates within and destroys helper T cells; in so doing, it seriously depresses the immune system. This depression elim-

inates the body's response to infection by fungi, protozoa, and other agents. The cell destruction also limits the ability of the body's B cells to produce antibodies. When the immune system is depressed, opportunistic illnesses and cancers develop.

Under normal circumstances, the body possesses about 800 to 1000 helper T cells per cubic millimeter of blood. As the destruction of T cells continues, the count drops over a period of weeks, months, or years, depending on a number of factors we will discuss. Profound immune deficiency occurs when the count drops below 100 cells per cubic millimeter.

Understanding the role of dendritic cells in HIV infection is also important to understanding how HIV spreads in the body. Dendritic cells are highly branched cells of the spleen and other lymphoid organs. The cells have long cytoplasmic extensions where antigens are engulfed for transport to the immune system. They may be among the first cells targeted by HIV following transmission through the body surface, most likely during sexual activity. Dendritic cells represent about 1 percent of the total white blood cell pool. Scientists have found that dendritic cells and helper T cells unite to form huge cells in which HIV reproduces.

Viremia

Viremia refers to a filling of the blood and tissues with infectious viruses. Primary HIV infection is associated with a burst of viremia. In many cases there is an accompanying abrupt decline of CD4+ T cells (helper T cells) in the peripheral blood as well. Figure 4.1 shows this pattern. The decrease in circulating T cells is probably due both to HIV-mediated killing of

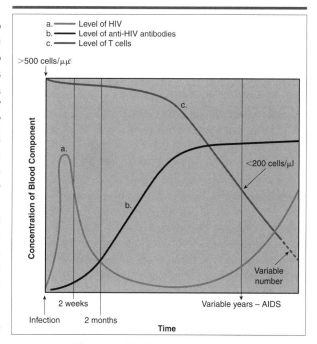

FIGURE 4.1 The dynamics of HIV, anti-HIV antibodies, and T cells over the course of HIV infection and AIDS.

cells and to redirection of T cells to the lymphoid tissues and other organs.

Early viral detection methods were insensitive to viral replication. The newer, more sensitive tests have demonstrated that viral replication is active throughout the course of infection and that it proceeds at levels far higher than previously imagined. HIV replication has been directly linked to the T cell destruction and depletion. In addition, ongoing HIV replication in the face of an ineffective host response is probably responsible for the secondary manifestations of HIV disease, including wasting and dementia.

Beginning with the first cycles of the virus replication in a newly infected host, HIV infection results in progressive destruction of the population of CD4+ T cells that serve essential roles in the generation of host immune responses. The target cell of preference for HIV infection and depletion is determined by the identity of the cell surface molecule CD4. This molecule is recognized by the HIV envelope glycoprotein when the virus binds to and enters host cells to initiate the replication cycle, as discussed in Chapter 3.

Macrophages and their counterparts within the central nervous system, the microglial cells, also express cell surface CD4 molecules and therefore provide targets for HIV infection. Because macrophages are more resistant to the destructive consequences of HIV infection than are T cells, their depletion is not quite so obvious. Also, as macrophages are widely distributed throughout the body, they probably serve an important role in persistent HIV infection by providing reservoirs of chronically infected cells.

The importance of the lymphoid organs in infected patients has been highlighted by the finding that concentrations of HIV-infected T cells are substantially higher in lymph nodes than in the peripheral blood. Thus, although the depletion of T cells after HIV infection is most readily revealed by sampling peripheral blood, the actual damage to the immune system is exacted in the lymphoid organs throughout the body. For example, the thymus is an early target of HIV infection and damage. This damage limits T cell production, especially in younger persons where thymus production of T cells is active.

In general terms, HIV infection compromises the source of helper T cells; this means the rate of the cell replenishment cannot continue indefinitely to match the rate of cell destruction. Consequently, T cell numbers decline in HIV-infected persons, both adults and children. After initial infection, the pace at which immune deficiency develops and the susceptibility to opportunistic illnesses are both associated with the rate of T cell decline. The decline differs considerably from person to person and is not constant throughout all stages of infection. Acceleration in the rate of T cell destruction heralds the progression of disease. Physicians often see increasing rates of HIV replication and the emergence of viruses demonstrating increased cytopathic effects for T cells together with

declining host cell-mediated immune response.

The progression of HIV disease is most readily gauged by declining T cell numbers. Research evidence indicates that the loss of specific types of immune responses also takes place. For example, memory T cells, which function in long-term immunity, are known to be preferred targets for HIV infection, and the loss of these cells is observed in HIV-infected persons even before substantial decreases are noted in other types of T cells. A gradual attrition of T cells depletes the repertoire of immune responses that can be effectively mounted. And this depletion predisposes a host to infection with opportunistic illnesses, as we shall explore presently.

 ## The Incubation Period

Host factors such as age or genetic differences among individuals may affect the incubation period, which is the time between entry of HIV to the host and the fulfillment of the case definition for AIDS. During this period, HIV is replicating in the body's helper T cells, but there are no physiologic responses to this replication. Thus, the infected individual exhibits no outward appearance that infection has taken place.

The median period of time between infection with HIV and the onset of clinically apparent disease is approximately 10 years in Western countries, according to prospective studies of men who have sex with men. The studies are based on cases where antibody tests have been performed on specific dates, that is, where dates of seroconversion are known ("seroconversion" refers to a positive HIV antibody test.) Similar estimates of asymptomatic periods have been made for HIV-infected blood transfusion recipients, injection drug users, and adult hemophiliacs.

However, HIV disease is not uniformly expressed in all individuals. A small proportion of persons infected with the virus develop AIDS and succumb within months following primary infection. Approximately 5 percent of individuals exhibit no signs of disease progression after 12 or more years; such individuals are referred to as long-term nonprogressors.

Other factors such as the virulence of the individual strain of virus and the presence of coinfection with other microorganisms may determine the rate and severity of HIV disease expression. These variables have been called clinical illness cofactors. They appear to influence the onset of disease among those infected with any pathogen. Cofactors are an important consideration in diseases such as hepatitis B and HIV infection. As disease progresses, the increasing amounts of infectious virus correlate with the worsening clinical course of disease. Studies in adults and children have shown that the levels of infectious HIV or proviral DNA in the blood are substantially higher in patients with AIDS than in asymptomatic patients.

Several mechanisms of CD4+ T cell killing have been observed in the laboratory, as discussed in Chapter 3, and they may explain the progressive loss of cells in HIV-infected individuals. These mechanisms include disruption of the cell membrane and the intracellular accumulation of viral-associated RNA and DNA molecules. The direct HIV-mediated cytopathic effect, and the formation of syncytia (sin-sish'ee-ah) also contribute to cell death. A syncytium (sin-sish'ee-um) is a giant cell that results when infected cells unite into a formless, functionless cell mass. The programmed death of cells, called apoptosis (a-po-to'sis), is another possible mode of cell death, as Chapter 3 explores.

Acute Primary HIV Infection

With acute primary HIV infection, a new phase of infection ensues. This is a short period of symptoms. The infected individual experiences a flu-like syndrome accompanied by malaise, fever, swollen lymph nodes, and occasionally a skin rash. A mononucleosis-like syndrome may occur as well, with mild fever, muscle aches and pains, and sore throat. Other symptoms are listed in Table 4.1.

During this period, involvement of the nervous system may lead to difficulty in concentrating, solving problems, or memory lapses. Convulsions and mental impairment may be experienced in extreme cases. An antibody test will be positive during this phase, and the patient will seroconvert (i.e., have a positive HIV antibody test). Transmission of the virus can occur during this phase as well as during the incubation period. Unfortunately, many individuals do not view these symptoms as signs of HIV infection, and they fail to seek diagnostic tests for HIV infection.

Period of Asymptomatic Infection

The period of acute primary HIV infection lasts only for a few days, then the symptoms disappear. Indeed, some individuals fail to develop acute primary HIV infection. A somewhat prolonged period of asymptomatic infection follows. It can last for several months or as long as 15 to 20 years. Behaviors to maintain health, such as exercising, can extend the time. Therapy to interrupt opportunistic illnesses before they begin can also extend the time, as Chapter 9 discusses. During this interval, antibodies can be demonstrated in the bloodstream, and HIV is also detectable in the blood at this stage. Its presence is noted by the viral load test that is described in Chapter 8. However, it should be pointed out that there are no clear symptoms of disease in this stage, and the level of circulating HIV is generally low.

During the prolonged asymptomatic period, a balance has been reached between the body's immune system and the infecting HIV. Helper T cells (i.e., CD4+ cells) are being produced to replace those lost, and transmission of the virus is possible. The existence of underlying health problems, such as tuberculosis, will hasten the progression to AIDS. For this reason it is important to identify the HIV-infected individual through one or more diagnostic procedures.

TABLE 4.1 Symptoms and Characteristics of Acute Primary HIV Infection

Clinical*

1. Headache, retro-orbital pain, muscle aches, sore throat, low-grade or high-grade fever, swollen lymph nodes
2. Nonpruritic macular erythematous rash
3. Oral candidiasis and ulcerations of the esophagus or anal canal
4. Acute central nervous system disorders (e.g., encephalitis)
5. Pneumonia
6. Diarrhea and other gastrointestinal complaints

Course

1. Symptoms last from 1 to 3 weeks
2. Lymphadenopathy, lethargy, and malaise can persist for many months
3. Generally followed by an asymptomatic period of months to years

Laboratory Findings

1. First week, lymphopenia and thrombocytopenia
2. Second week, lymphocyte number rises secondary to an increase in number of CD8+ cells; CD4/CD8 ratio decreases
3. Second week, atypical lymphocytes appear in the blood (generally <50%)
4. HIV antigenemia and viremia detected
5. Virus might be present in cerebrospinal fluid and in seminal fluid
6. Anti-HIV antibodies first detected within 6 to 14 days

*Some or all of these findings may be present.

Generalized Lymphadenopathy

The Centers for Disease Control and Prevention (CDC) has established a case definition for individuals with HIV infection, as outlined in Table 4.2. This case definition generally implies the presence of a wasting syndrome, dementia, or opportunistic illness. But before any of these ensues, the patient enters a preliminary phase during which the symptoms of immune suppression become obvious.

The phase is referred to as generalized lymphadenopathy (lim-fad-eh-nop'ah-thee). It results from the immune system's failure to defend against HIV, and the replication of HIV within infected cells. The lymph nodes are persistently swollen and rubbery. The patient experiences a constant low-grade fever, night sweats, continuous or intermittent diarrhea, and unexplained weight loss. Fatigue becomes substantial, memory lapses are common, and the patient experiences the "blues." These symptoms generally indicate that progression to AIDS is imminent.

In past years, the CDC has used the term "AIDS-related complex" (ARC) for all the stages leading up to AIDS. This term is used less often now; instead, the patient is said to have HIV infection during any of the infection periods discussed previously. The next stage is now referred to simply as AIDS.

TABLE 4.2 The CDC Classification System for HIV Infection

	Clinical Categories		
CD4+ T Cell Categories	**A** **Asymptomatic, Acute (Primary) HIV or PGL**	**B** **Symptomatic, Not (A) or (C) Conditions**	**C** **AIDS-Indicator Conditions**
(1) ≥500/mm^3	A1	B1	C1
(2) 200–499/mm^3	A2	B2	C2
(3) <200/mm^3 AIDS-indicator T cell count	A3	B3	C3

Clinical Categories of HIV

Category A:
One or more of the conditions listed below in an adolescent or adult (≥13 years) with documented HIV infection. Conditions listed in Categories B and C must not have occurred.
- Asymptomatic HIV infection
- Persistent generalized lymphadenopathy
- Acute (primary) HIV infection with accompanying illness or history of acute HIV infection

Category B:
Symptomatic conditions in an HIV-infected adolescent or adult that are not included among conditions listed in clinical Category C and that meet at least one of the following criteria: a. the conditions are attributed to HIV infection or are indicative of a defect in cell-mediated immunity; or b. the conditions are considered by physicians to have a clinical course or to require management that is complicated by HIV infection. **Examples** of conditions in clinical Category B include, **but are not limited to:**
- Bacillary angiomatosis
- Candidiasis, oropharyngeal (thrush)
- Candidiasis, vulvovaginal; persistent, frequent, or poorly responsive to therapy
- Cervical dysplasia (moderate or severe)/cervical carcinoma in situ
- Constitutional symptoms, such as fever (38.5°C) or diarrhea lasting >1 month
- Herpes zoster (shingles), involving at least two distinct episodes or more than one dermatome
- Idiopathic thrombocytopenic purpura
- Listeriosis
- Pelvic inflammatory disease, particularly if complicated by tubo-ovarian abscess
- Peripheral neuropathy

For classification purposes, Category B conditions take precedence over those in Category A. For example, someone previously treated for oral or persistent vaginal candidiasis (and who has not developed a Category C disease) but who is now asymptomatic should be classified in clinical Category B.

Category C:
Includes the clinical conditions listed in the AIDS surveillance case definition. For classification purposes, once a Category C condition has occurred, the person will remain in Category C.

In previous years, this next stage was referred to as "full-blown AIDS," another term that is no longer used.

 ## The Case Definition for AIDS

For surveillance purposes, the CDC currently defines AIDS in an adult or adolescent (age 13 years or older) as the presence of 1 or more of the 25 AIDS-indicator conditions. Table 4.3 lists these conditions, which include Kaposi's sarcoma, *Pneumocystis* pneumonia, or other opportunistic illnesses. In children younger than 13 years the definition of AIDS is similar to that for adolescents and adults, except that recurrent bacterial illnesses are included in the list of the AIDS-defining conditions. In 1993 the case definition for adults and adolescents was expanded to include HIV infection in an individual with a CD4+ T cell count of less than 200 cells per cubic millimeter of blood. This current surveillance definition replaces the 1987 criteria, which were based on clinical conditions and evidence of HIV infection but not on helper T cell determinations.

These criteria have been established to ensure unity in the reporting of cases of AIDS, and the CDC definition should be used by all individuals having anything to do with AIDS. Surveillance definitions are epidemiologically useful for tracking and quantifying the epidemic and its manifestations. In clinical practice, the symptoms and measurements of immune function, notably the levels of CD4+ T cells, are used to guide treatment of HIV-infected persons. AIDS represents the end stage of a continuous, progressive pathogenic process;

it begins with primary infection with HIV, continues with a chronic phase that is usually without symptoms, leads to progressively severe symptoms, and ultimately results in profound immunodeficiency with opportunistic illnesses and neoplasms, as described below. The breakdown of the immune system of HIV-infected patients goes on gradually over a long period of time, but eventually most individuals with HIV infection will progress to AIDS.

Progression to AIDS

The progression to AIDS comes as the T cell count approaches 200 per cubic millimeter. Now the patient begins to experience oral lesions such as hairy leukoplakia (lu-koh-play'kee-ah). Other oral diseases at this stage may include canker sores from herpes viruses, and thrush caused by the fungus *Candida albicans*. Neuropathologies such as loss of motor control and peripheral numbness are also reported. Cognitive slowing may also occur.

When the T cell count is about 200 per cubic millimeter of blood, the HIV-infected individual is likely to experience opportunistic illnesses. For this reason, the case definition for AIDS includes a helper T cell count of 200 per cubic millimeter or less. Opportunistic illnesses may occur in the lungs, gastrointestinal tract, and skin. Immune suppression allows normally benign illnesses to deteriorate to severe disease if not treated promptly.

Patient education will help the individual avoid opportunistic illnesses, as we will discuss presently. Stress

TABLE 4.3 Some of the Opportunistic Illnesses Associated with AIDS

Pathogen or Disease	Disease Description
Protozoa	
Pneumocystis carinii	Life-threatening pneumonia
Cryptosporidium	Persistent diarrhea
Toxoplasma gondii	Encephalitis
Isospora belli	Gastroenteritis
Viruses	
Cytomegalovirus	Fever, encephalitis, blindness
Herpes simplex virus	Vesicles of skin and mucous membranes
Varicella-zoster virus	Shingles
Fungi	
Histoplasma capsulatum	Disseminated infection
Cryptococcus neoformans	Disseminated, but especially meningitis
Candida albicans	Overgrowth on oral and vaginal mucous membranes (Category B stage of HIV infection)
	Overgrowth in esophagus, lungs (Category C stage of HIV infection)
Cancers or Precancerous Conditions	
Kaposi's sarcoma	Cancer of skin and blood vessels (probably caused by a herpesvirus)
Hairy leukoplakia	Whitish patches on mucous membranes; commonly considered precancerous
Cervical dysplasia	Abnormal cervical growth

reduction, good nutritional habits, exercise, and other health-ful behaviors can also be encouraged. Instruction on avoiding transmission of virus to others is also paramount. Antiviral therapy will be recommended, if it has not already begun. Antidepression education will also be helpful.

As the T cell count continues to fall, the patient becomes more susceptible to opportunistic illnesses and conditions that may be life-threatening. Because the individual now has AIDS, a psychological change occurs, and depression is likely. Social stigmas will be felt, and assistance in the day-to-day activities of normal living will become more important to the patient.

As the count of T cells drops below 50 per cubic millime-ter, the patient is probably experiencing an AIDS-related opportunistic illness at all times. Multiple medications may be required, as well as antiretroviral therapy. There is a constant need to deal with symptoms, and the severe discomfort involves psychological as well as physical stress. Emaciation and uncontrollable diarrhea often occur. Social interaction is commonly reduced and fatigue is constant. The involvement of the caregiver at this stage is significant, and will continue to be more important as the disease progresses.

Several classifications have been used to establish the progression of signs and symptoms from HIV infection to AIDS. Developed to provide a framework for the medical man-agement of the disease, the classification systems are funda-mentally similar. One classification called the Walter Reed Army Medical Center System establishes six stages for pro-gression (Table 4.4). A second classification established by the CDC uses four groupings exclusive of one another. The groups are important to individuals having direct involvement with the disease and to the organizations who gather statistics. They provide representative indicators so that HIV can be tracked during its progression to AIDS.

Children with AIDS, experience reduced cognitive skills, probably because HIV has invaded the brain tissue. The chil-dren fail to thrive. Their growth patterns are interrupted, and they suffer substantial loss of weight or fail to gain weight.

Diarrhea tends to be persistent, and intelligence milestones are not reached. Many of the opportunistic illnesses experi-enced by adults also occur in children.

Opportunistic Illnesses

Because of the suppression of the immune system, individuals infected by HIV are susceptible to a broad variety of illnesses caused by opportunistic microorganisms. Some of these organisms normally exist in a benign state in the body as the immune system keeps them in check. However, when the sys-tem is repressed, the organisms seize the "opportunity" and invade the tissues. In many individuals, the opportunistic microorganisms are the cause of death in the individual who has HIV infection. Moreover, their presence is a sign that the individual has AIDS or another condition involving immuno-suppression. Diseases caused by opportunistic microorgan-isms are referred to as opportunistic illnesses.

Protozoa   Over half the deaths associated with AIDS are caused by infection with a protozoan called *Pneumocystis carinii*. This statistic is shown in Table 4.5, where the per-centages of decedent men in three categories is compared to the disease they died from.

Some researchers classify *Pneumocystis carinii* as a fun-gus because of its biochemical constituents, but we will refer to it as a protozoan because its structure, life cycle, and phys-iological characteristics are similar to other protozoa. The organism is present in the dormant state in the lungs of most individuals in the United States. Before the AIDS epidemic, the organism was associated with immune suppressing treat-ments. However since the beginning of the AIDS epidemic, *Pneumocystis carinii* has been recognized as the cause of the most prevalent opportunistic illness in patients infected with HIV.

Pneumocystis carinii causes an insidious pneumonia. Patients experience a shortness of breath and substantial dam-age to the lungs. The organisms multiply in the lung tissue and cause consolidation so that gas exchange cannot take

TABLE 4.4   The Walter Reed AMC Classification System for the Progression to AIDS

Stage	HIV Antibody and/or Virus	Chronic Lymphadenopathy	Helper T-Lymphocytes per mm³	Delayed Hypersensitivity	Thrush	Opportunistic Diseases
WR0	−	−	>400	NORMAL	−	−
WR1	+	−	>400	NORMAL	−	−
WR2	+	+	>400	NORMAL	−	−
WR3	+	+/−	<400	NORMAL	−	−
WR4	+	+/−	<400	P	−	−
WR5	+	+/−	<400	P/C	+/−	−
WR6	+	+/−	<400	P/C	+/−	+

Note: P, partial reaction; P/C, partial or complete reaction; +/−, may or may not occur.

TABLE 4.5 Percentage of Men in Three Categories Who Died of a Given Opportunistic Illness, 1992–1997

Disease	Total (N = 8811)	Men Who Have Sex with Men (N = 5168)	Injection Drug Users (N = 1520)	Males Exposed to HIV Through Heterosexual Contact (N = 243)
Pneumocystis carinii pneumonia	52.8	52.1	52.9	45.0
Mycobacterium avium complex	30.2	31.7	19.2	22.7
Esophageal candidiasis	24.1	23.5	28.1	24.4
Kaposi's sarcoma	23.8	27.4	4.1	5.4
Cytomegalovirus retinitis	21.3	24.2	6.7	11.9
Wasting syndrome	20.8	20.9	22.8	19.6
HIV encephalopathy	11.6	13.8	9.2	13.1
Cytomegalovirus disease	13.4	15.4	3.0	2.5
Extrapulmonary cryptococcosis	8.1	7.6	9.0	13.9
Recurrent pneumonia	7.2	6.9	9.0	13.0
Toxoplasmosis of brain	7.1	6.8	10.6	13.0
Pulmonary tuberculosis	6.4	4.8	18.5	13.5
Chronic cryptosporidiosis	6.0	6.6	2.3	4.7
Chronic herpes simplex	4.7	4.6	4.0	5.1
Extrapulmonary tuberculosis	4.0	3.2	9.0	5.3
Other disseminated *Mycobacterium*	3.3	3.6	2.4	1.5
Immunoblastic lymphoma	3.1	3.4	1.5	1.3
Progressive Multifocal leukoencephalopathy	2.7	2.9	2.2	2.0
Primary brain lymphoma	2.2	2.4	1.0	1.0
Disseminated histoplasmosis	1.6	1.6	1.8	1.9
Pulmonary candidiasis	1.0	1.1	1.0	0.7
Burkitt's lymphoma	0.9	1.1	0.1	0.4
Disseminated coccidioidomycosis	0.2	0.2	0.0	0.4
Recurrent *Salmonella* septicemia	0.2	0.2	0.4	1.1
Chronic isosporiasis	0.1	0.1	0.0	0.0

place. Fever, dry cough, and shortness of breath accompany the infection. Over 80 percent of AIDS patients develop *P. carinii* pneumonia (PCP) at some time, and in over 35 percent of men, it is the first opportunistic illness to occur. (Table 4.6 compares the first instance of this and other opportunistic illnesses in men.) Chest X rays show the characteristic growth in both right and left lung, and the organism can be seen on microscopic examination of washings from the respiratory tract.

For those having a positive test for HIV, *Pneumocystis* pneumonia can be prevented by inhaling the drug pentamidine (pen-tam'i-deen) isethionate (i-se-thi'o-nate). This drug can also be used by those who have active illnesses. Sulfa drugs such as sulfamethoxazole (sul"-fa-meth-ok'sah-zole) combined with trimethoprim (tri-meth'oh-prim) are also effective and in some cases, they are preferred to pentamidine because the side effects are less powerful.

Another protozoan causing opportunistic illness is *Toxoplasma gondii*. This organism causes a brain inflammation called toxoplasmosis (tox-so-plaz-mo'sis). Cats are often infected with this organism (although no symptoms are seen), so people with HIV infection are encouraged to avoid these animals or to restrict their time out of doors, as Chapter 6 indicates. Seizures commonly occur in infected individuals. In uninfected adults, a mononucleosis-like infection may occur with few symptoms, but in AIDS patients the brain inflammation is similar to viral encephalitis (en-sef-ah-li'tis). The symptoms resemble those seen with brain tumors, and convulsions and dementia occur. Antibiotics such as sulfadiazine (sul-fa-di'ah-zeen) and pyrimethamine (pir-i-meth'ah-meen) are used in treatment.

Still another protozoal infection is caused by *Cryptosporidium parvum* and other species of *Cryptosporidium* (krip"-to-spor-id'i-um). This organism causes cryptosporidiosis (krip"-to-spor-id-i-o'sis), with diarrhea that is extraordinarily excessive and unrelenting. Mild diarrhea occurs in healthy adults, but in AIDS patients it is severe and prolonged. Indeed, the AIDS patient may experience over 25 watery stools per day accompanied by cramping and weight loss. The electrolyte (salt) balance of the body and the nutri-

TABLE 4.6 Percentage of Men in Three Categories In Whom a Given Opportunistic Illness Occurred First, 1992–1997

Disease	Total (N = 10,658)	Men Who Have Sex with Men (N = 5964)	Injection Drug Users (N = 1865)	Males Exposed to HIV Through Heterosexual Contact (N = 372)
Pneumocystis carinii pneumonia	35.7	34.6	35.6	35.1
Kaposi's sarcoma	12.5	15.0	2.0	3.7
Esophageal candidiasis	11.9	11.0	15.5	15.2
Wasting syndrome	7.8	7.7	10.6	6.9
Mycobacterium avium complex	6.4	6.6	6.2	9.5
Pulmonary tuberculosis	4.8	3.1	13.7	8.1
Extrapulmonary cryptococcosis	4.3	4.0	4.4	4.6
HIV encephalopathy	4.2	4.3	3.3	3.2
Cytomegalovirus retinitis	3.8	4.4	1.6	1.6
Cytomegalovirus disease	3.4	4.1	0.9	0.7
Toxoplasmosis of brain	2.9	2.3	6.7	5.1
Chronic cryptosporidiosis	2.9	3.3	0.7	1.1
Recurrent pneumonia	2.3	1.8	4.9	5.0
Extrapulmonary tuberculosis	2.0	1.6	4.6	4.6
Chronic herpes simplex	2.0	1.9	1.6	2.9
Immunoblastic lymphoma leukoencephalopathy	1.6	1.9	0.7	0.7
Progressive multifocal leukoencephalopathy	1.1	1.2	0.8	0.9
Disseminated histoplasmosis	0.7	0.7	0.9	2.1
Burkitt's lymphoma	0.7	1.0	0.0	0.5
Other disseminated *Mycobacterium*	0.6	0.6	0.8	0.3
Primary brain lymphoma	0.4	0.5	0.4	0.0
Pulmonary candidiasis	0.3	0.2	0.8	0.3
Disseminated coccidioidomycosis	0.1	0.1	0.1	0.4
Recurrent *Salmonella* septicemia	0.1	0.1	0.3	0.4
Chronic isosporiasis	0.0	0.0	0.0	0.0

tional patterns become profoundly disturbed. Although it does not occurr in most AIDS patients, cryptosporidiosis can be severe and occasionally lethal. Other protozoa cause infections in AIDS patients as well, including *Isospora belli* (intestinal infection) and *Microsporidium* (intestinal infection).

Fungi   Among the fungi that live in the body, several organisms can cause serious infections in the HIV-infected individual. One of the most commonly encountered is *Candida albicans*, the agent of thrush (technically known as mucocutaneous candidiasis, (mu"-co-cu-tan'e-ous can-di-di'a-sis). This disease involves an overgrowth of *C. albicans* in the oral cavity and down into the esophagus. It is one of the first signs that AIDS has begun. The fungus is depicted in Figure 4.2.

Candida albicans is normally found in the mouth without any complication, but in the AIDS patient it will grow profusely and invade the esophageal lining, causing erosion and exposing the nerve fibers. The AIDS patient cannot swallow without pain, and the desire to eat is soon lost. Furry

white plaques occur in the mouth, but antifungal drugs can control them up to a point. *Candida albicans* infection is often a persistent problem throughout the time during which AIDS is present. Systemic infection can occur as well.

Among the fungi infecting the internal organs is *Cryptococcus* (krip'-toh-kok'us) *neoformans*. The fungus enters the lung, then passes to the bloodstream and brain where it causes a severe brain disease known as cryptococcosis (krip"-toh-kok-oh'sis). The spinal cord is involved in many cases, and a fatal paralytic disease may ensue. Pneumonia, kidney disease, and bone marrow disease are other complications of illnesses with this fungus. A drug called amphotericin B is used in therapy, but the infection tends to be extremely aggressive. The organism is present in the dropping of pigeons, so AIDS patients are advised to avoid areas where these birds tend to flock.

Other key fungi significant in AIDS are *Histoplasma capsulatum* (his-to-plaz'mah cap-su-la'tum) and *Coccidioides immitis* (kok-sid-i-oi'-dez im'mi-tis). Both fungi occasionally cause lung disease in healthy individuals, but in the AIDS

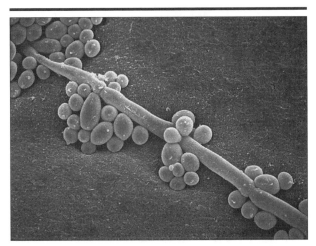

FIGURE 4.2   An electron micrograph of *Candida albicans*, a yeastlike fungus that causes esophageal and other infections in a person with AIDS.

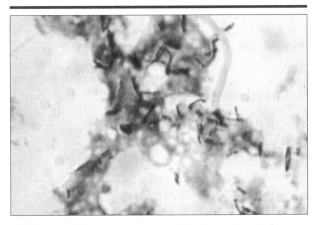

FIGURE 4.3   A light micrograph of *Mycobacterium tuberculosis*, the cause of tuberculosis. This acid-fast rod causes serious lung disease in the AIDS patient.

patient, the fungi cause severe pneumonia before infecting the entire body. Amphotericin B can be used for treatment. These fungi are abundant in certain parts of the United States, and AIDS patients may be advised to restrict their travel to these sections of the country. For example, *C. immitis* exists widely in the southwestern United States.

Bacteria   Numerous bacteria are able to cause infection in the HIV-infected individual. Among the most aggressive is *Mycobacterium tuberculosis*, shown in Figure 4.3. This organism is a bacterial rod that causes tuberculosis in healthy individuals as well as in immune suppressed individuals. Once it is established in one section of the lung, *M. tuberculosis* then spreads throughout the chest cavity, causing a progressive and sustained destruction of the lungs. The chest X ray displays numerous patches of lung infections. The patient expels rust-colored sputum from the pulmonary tract, and, as

the breathing becomes labored, the patient often becomes unable to catch his or her breath.

In today's world, tuberculosis is a major health problem of global proportions. Hundreds of millions of individuals are believed infected by the organism. The superimposition of the tuberculosis epidemic with the AIDS epidemic has created a problem of massive proportions for public heath agencies. Although drugs are available to control tuberculosis (e.g., isoniazid, rifampin, ethambutol, and others), public health agencies face a burdensome task of dealing with the two epidemics.

Another species of *Mycobacterium* known as *Mycobacterium avium-intracellulare* (a'vee-um in"-tra-cell-u-lar'ay) causes a tuberculosis-like infection of the lungs. Often known as MAI disease, the opportunistic illness is common during late stages of immunosuppression and is often a cause of death in AIDS patients.

Another bacterium responsible for respiratory disease in infected individuals is *Streptococcus pneumoniae*, which causes pneumococcal pneumonia. In addition, many species of the Gram-negative rod *Salmonella* are known to cause infection of the gastrointestinal tract during all stages of infection. Another bacterium of concern is *Shigella*, a Gram-negative rod that causes of serious form of diarrhea known as shigellosis (shi-gel-o'sis). In AIDS patients, the common bacterium *Staphylococcus aureus* can cause severe skin disease, but topical antibiotics can be used to control these infections.

Viruses   Of course the most important virus associated with AIDS is HIV. Apart from this virus, however, others can also occur in the infected individual. Among the most common viruses causing problems is the cytomegalovirus (si-to-meg'a-lo-virus). This member of the herpesvirus family causes severe infection of the eye, especially the retina, and infected patients often develop blindness. The drug ganciclovir (gan-ci'clo-vir) is available to treat the disease, but the drug has toxic side effects. The cytomegalovirus also causes pneumonia, diarrhea, and skin rashes in infected individuals.

Another herpesvirus known as the varicella-zoster (VZ) virus causes shingles in the HIV-infected individual. Shingles are exquisitely sensitive and highly painful blisters and lesions occurring around the body trunk and sometimes on the face and scalp. Many individuals harbor this virus as a result of an early bout of chickenpox, and HIV appears to trigger the virus to infect, but this time as shingles. Outbreaks of herpes simplex are also seen in numerous HIV-infected persons.

Many individuals develop a condition of the mouth called hairy leukoplakia, as noted earlier. In this condition, the papillae (pap-il'ae) cells of the tongue become abnormally large and produce plaques with cells that resemble cancer cells. The Epstein-Barr virus (a cause of infectious mononucleosis) is believed to stimulate this condition. Hairy leukoplakia is not completely understood at this writing but appears to be unique to AIDS patients.

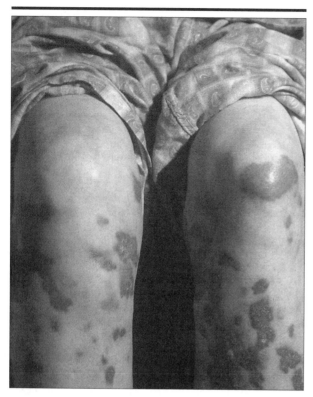

FIGURE 4.4 A patient showing the skin lesions associated with Kaposi's sarcoma, an opportunistic illness in persons with AIDS.

Cancer An abnormal growth of cells that forms a tumor then spreads is a cancer. The most prevalent cancer associated with AIDS is Kaposi's sarcoma. Believed to be caused by a herpesvirus, Kaposi's sarcoma is a virulent disease in AIDS patients. It is accompanied by painless, flat and raised, pink to purplish plaques on the skin and mucosal surfaces at the body orifices, as shown in Figure 4.4. The plaques develop in many internal organs including the liver, spleen, blood vessels, lung, and parts of the gastrointestinal tract. In AIDS patients, the disease spreads aggressively and rapidly—much more aggressively than the classic form of Kaposi's sarcoma, which is a slow developing and relatively painless disease. Several chemical agents are now available to slow the progression of the tumors, and in many cases therapy can eliminate them completely.

Another cancer affecting AIDS patients is lymphoma (lim-pho'ma). This is a cancer of the B cells of the lymphoid tissue. Although it is relatively rare in AIDS patients, it has been seen among those having persistent swelling of the lymph nodes. Confusion, memory loss, and neurological symptoms often accompany the disease because the lymphomas occur in the brain tissue.

Cancer and other opportunistic illnesses are the major cause of morbidity and mortality among persons infected with HIV. However, as a result of new treatments that improve out-

comes for HIV-infected persons, the prevalence of persons who live with AIDS and opportunistic illnesses is increasing. In 1997, over 271,000 persons were living with AIDS in the United States and were at high risk for contracting opportunistic illnesses. In 1997, over 21,000 HIV-infected persons died from the effects of AIDS, nearly all from opportunistic illnesses. Figure 4.5 summarizes the many body organs affected by the opportunistic illnesses and lists some illnesses not discussed above.

Other AIDS-Associated Illnesses

HIV affects the body in other locales as well as in the immune system. For example, scientists now know that HIV infects the brain tissue, causing neurological disease. Entry to the brain is probably related to phagocytic white blood cells called monocytes. Monocytes become various types of specialized cells including macrophages. When the macrophages develop into microglial cells within the brain, they carry HIV across the blood-brain barrier and thereby permit HIV to enter the brain tissue.

Many patients suffer AIDS-associated dementia. A progressive series of symptoms appears, including loss of mental function, difficulty in reasoning, depression, and personality changes. In the most severe cases, patients are unable to care for themselves and resemble those suffering from Alzheimer's disease. Spinal cord damage and peripheral nerve damage may also occur.

Some AIDS patients suffer a wasting syndrome as HIV causes a continuing loss in body weight. Uncontrolled diarrhea often accompanies this wasting, and the patient may lose over 10 percnet of the total body weight. Although the pathology of this syndrome is not totally explained by the infection process and is not completely understood, it is widespread in AIDS patients. High fevers, usually experienced as night sweats accompany the wasting.

The relationship between immune system depression, wasting, and nervous system involvement in AIDS patients may be explained by the relationship between the immune and nervous systems. In recent years, scientists have discovered that helper T cells respond to the presence of neuropeptides (neu-ro-pep'tides), a series of stress hormones released by the adrenal glands in response to messages from the brain. Research indicates that some T cells manufacture their own peptides. Also, the secretions of activated T cells can transmit information to the brain. In addition, thymus hormones act on brain cells.

The data indicate that the immune system may exert a direct influence on the brain and may be directed, at least in part, by secretions from the brain. Networks of nerve fibers have been found connecting regions within the lymphoid organs, further evidence of a relationship between the systems. Thus, the destruction of the immune system's helper T cells may affect not only the immune system, but also the

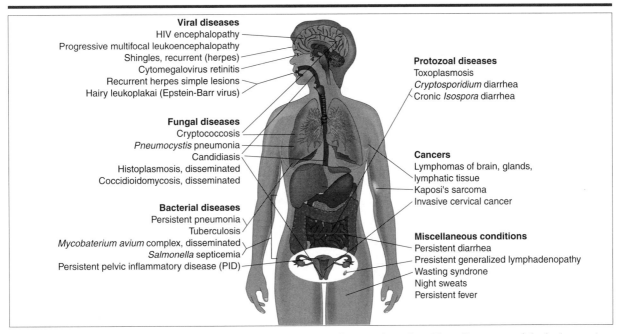

Viral diseases
HIV encephalopathy
Progressive multifocal leukoencephalopathy
Shingles, recurrent (herpes)
Cytomegalovirus retinitis
Recurrent herpes simple lesions
Hairy leukoplakai (Epstein-Barr virus)

Fungal diseases
Cryptococcosis
Pneumocystis pneumonia
Candidiasis
Histoplasmosis, disseminated
Coccidioidomycosis, disseminated

Bacterial diseases
Persistent pneumonia
Tuberculosis
Mycobaterium avium complex, disseminated
Salmonella septicemia
Persistent pelvic inflammatory disease (PID)

Protozoal diseases
Toxoplasmosis
Cryptosporidium diarrhea
Cronic *Isospora* diarrhea

Cancers
Lymphomas of brain, glands, lymphatic tissue
Kaposi's sarcoma
Invasive cervical cancer

Miscellaneous conditions
Persistent diarrhea
Presistent generalized lymphadenopathy
Wasting syndrone
Night sweats
Persistent fever

FIGURE 4.5 The various regions of the body and the opportunistic illnesses they affect. Virtually no part of the body remains unaffected of these illnesses.

nervous system. The wasting syndrome may be yet another manifestation of the brain's interaction with the body, following an interruption of the immune system functioning.

Still another effect of HIV on the body involves interruption of macrophage function. Macrophages are large white blood cells that perform phagocytosis, as noted in Chapter 2 and above. They mingle among the body tissues and interact with and ingest bacteria, fungi, protozoa, and other microorganisms. In doing so, they provide resistance to diseases. Researchers have found HIV within the macrophages of lung tissues in AIDS patients. The viruses multiply within membranous compartments of the cells, and thereby escape cellular defenses. When such an infection takes place, the macrophages cannot produce the messages that activate CD4+ cells (helper T cells). This action further blocks the immune response from taking place. Indeed, in some individuals the T cells appear to occur in normal number and condition, but during infection the macrophages may prevent the T cells from functioning.

In addition, macrophages may serve as a reservoir for HIV in the body. Macrophages are relatively resistant to the destructive affects of HIV, and the virus survives in these cells and is transported to various other organs in the body. Thus, the macrophage may be a key intermediary in the spread of HIV infection.

 Perinatal AIDS

Perinatal transmission of HIV accounts for virtually all new HIV infections in children. As of 1993, an estimated 15,000 HIV-infected children had been born to HIV-positive women in the United States. Then, in 1994, clinical trials demonstrated a two-thirds reduction in the risk for perinatal transmission when treatment of HIV-infected pregnant women was instituted and when infants were treated with azidothymidine (AZT), also known as zidovudine (ZDV). Thereafter, a continued and substantial decline in the incidence of AIDS occurred in children who were infected through perinatal HIV transmission. As of mid-1999, perinatal transmission accounted for 8596 of the 711,344 total AIDS cases in adults and children—only one percent of the cases.

The estimated number of children with perinatal AIDS diagnosed each year declined 43 percent during the period of 1992 to 1996. The effectiveness of AZT therapy in reducing perinatal HIV transmission has thus been documented. The decline in perinatal HIV transmission highlights the effectiveness of and ongoing need for these treatment strategies:

• Ensuring that women receive adequate prenatal care, timely HIV counseling, and voluntary testing

• Giving women access to HIV-related care services

• Providing them with prophylaxis to reduce perinatal transmission

• Counseling mothers to avoid breast-feeding.

At the time of this writing, most HIV-infected children are born in developing countries. The United Nations Program on HIV estimates that each year of 350,000 children in developing countries are infected with HIV through perinatal transmission. The World Health Organization estimates

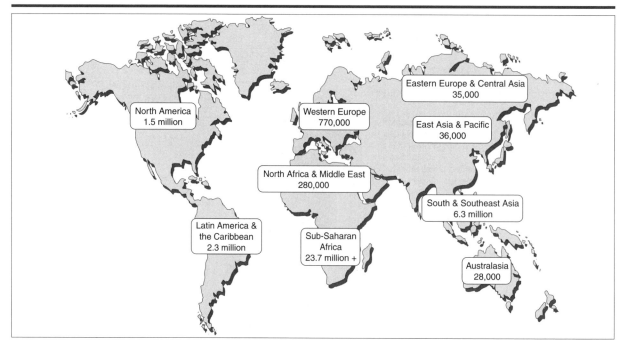

FIGURE 4.6   The World Health Organization's estimate of the numbers of persons living with HIV infection/AIDS as of early 1999. Reports have been made by 209 countries. Over 1 million of the cases have occurred in children.

that over 1 million children worldwide now have HIV infection (Figure 4.6 shows the figures for all individuals).

 HIV-2 and AIDS

In the mid-1990s, researchers reported that HIV-2 infection is less likely to cause a person to progress to AIDS than HIV-1. The study was done in female sex workers (prostitutes) in Senegal over a 10-year period. Investigators studied women infected with HIV-1 and contrasted their rate of progression to the rate of progression for women infected with HIV-2. Based on the statistics of progression, researchers at the Harvard AIDS Institute made the projection that women infected with HIV-1 have a 33% chance of developing AIDS within 5 years. However, women infected with HIV-2 have almost no chance of progressing to AIDS within the same five-year period.

HIV-2 is found mainly in West Africa, as well as India, Brazil, and some parts of Europe. It remains relatively rare in the United States. The principal mode of transmission of HIV-2 in West Africa is through sexual contact, although some cases are related to injection drug use or blood transfusions. The clinical course of HIV-2 infection is much slower than for HIV-1 and there seems to be a much longer incubation period. Over time, however, people become ill and develop a syndrome similar to that of classic HIV-1 infection. Figure 4.6 shows the enormous numbers of people worldwide who have HIV infection. HIV-2 accounts for a percentage of these cases.

In persons with HIV-2 infection who progress to AIDS, diarrheal illnesses related to intestinal pathogens are by far the most common opportunistic illnesses. Some individuals experience Kaposi's sarcoma as well as toxoplasmosis, candidiasis, tuberculosis, *Salmonella* infection, and herpes zoster. *Pneumocystis carinii* pneumonia is relatively rare. Despite the clinical differences, HIV-2 encodes many of the same gene products as HIV-1. However, the *vpu* gene is not found in HIV-2, and another gene, the *vpx* gene, is found in HIV-2 but not in HIV-1. As of 1992, the FDA has mandated that all blood donations be tested for HIV-2 as well as HIV-1.

Questions

1. Describe the host cells involved in the initial viremia that accompanies HIV infection.

2. Outline the case definition for AIDS and describe the period immediately preceding the progression to AIDS.

3. Name and summarize a series of opportunistic illnesses that occur in the AIDS patient.

Chapter Five

The Spreading AIDS Epidemic

Review and Preview

Thus far we have explored the concepts of disease and the resistance. We learned that infectious disease is a complex process of interactions between microbe and host; depending upon which prevails, the disease can take different courses. We showed that the immune system is the body's major way of reacting to infectious microorganisms, and we noted that interference with this system severely impedes the body's ability to resist disease.

Two separate branches of the immune system are responsible for antibody-mediated immunity and cell-mediated immunity, respectively. We noted that the human immunodeficiency virus (HIV) has a destructive effect on the branch leading to cell-mediated immunity because it destroys the helper T cells that underpin the system. We also described HIV as an RNA virus enclosed in the protein coat and an envelope containing spikes. The spikes contain two proteins designated gp120 and gp41, both used to facilitate union of the virus with cellular receptors at the surface of the T cell. Once this union has taken place, the nucleocapsid of the virus enters the cell, and reverse transcriptase synthesizes a DNA molecule that integrates to the cellular DNA in the nucleus. From that site, the DNA encodes the production of new HIV particles in the host T cell. During this process, the T cells are destroyed by cell membrane injury, by the formation of syncytia, or by the overwhelming parasitism of HIV.

In Chapter 4, the primary thrust was to illustrate how this destruction of T cells affects the body. We saw that the progression of HIV infection is gauged in part by declining T cell numbers. As the rate of T cell destruction accelerates, the individual with HIV infection progresses to acquired immune deficiency syndrome (AIDS). In Western countries, the median period of time between infection and the onset of clinically apparent disease is approximately 10 years, but some persons progress before that time and some progress later.

Before AIDS develops in an individual, the person may experience acute primary HIV infection, which is a short period of symptoms including a flu-like syndrome and possible nervous system involvement. A period of asymptomatic infection may follow, and generalized lymphadenopathy may then develop. The case definition for AIDS is fulfilled when the person has a T cell count of less than 200 cells per cubic millimeter of blood and when an opportunistic illness occurs.

Among the first opportunistic illnesses to appear is infection caused by the fungus *Candida albicans*. This fungus grows in the mouth and down the esophagus, where it erodes the esophageal lining, causing exposure of the nerve endings and very painful swallowing.

Over half the deaths associated with AIDS are caused by an opportunistic illness due to the protozoan *Pneumocystis carinii*. This organism causes an insidious pneumonia. Another protozoan, *Toxoplasma gondii*, causes a brain inflammation called toxoplasmosis. Still another protozoan, *Cryptosporidium*, causes an unrelenting diarrhea.

Numerous fungi, bacteria, and viruses cause opportunistic illnesses associated with AIDS. For example, the bacterium *Mycobacterium tuberculosis* commonly infects AIDS patients and causes tuberculosis, which begins in one lung and then spreads throughout the chest cavity resulting in a progressive and sustained deterioration of the tissues. The most common virus causing opportunistic illness is the cytomegalovirus. This virus causes severe infection of the eye, often resulting in blindness. The most prevalent cancer associated with AIDS is Kaposi's sarcoma. This disease is accompanied by painless, flat and raised, pink to purplish plaques on the skin and in many internal organs as well.

Paramount to dealing with AIDS is understanding how the disease spreads in the community. That will be the theme of this chapter as we explore the modes of sexual transmission, modes of blood transfusion, and mechanisms by which HIV moves from mothers to their unborn children. By familiarizing ourselves with these modes we can be better equipped to prevent the spread of AIDS and avoid the tortures that it afflicts on the body.

Introduction

AIDS has been the subject of intense inquiry since the disease was first identified as a clinical entity in 1981. More than any other medical problem of our era, AIDS poses a serious threat to humans for several reasons: recognizing the disease can be difficult; methods of treatment are generally ill-defined; complete cures are few or nonexistent; and the majority of infected individuals are in danger of dying.

Identifying how HIV moves from person to person is a subtopic of the science of epidemiology. Epidemiologists study the patterns of disease in populations and the factors affecting those patterns. Beginning in 1981 epidemiologists identified AIDS as a new syndrome and showed that it was occurring with high frequency in sexually active men who have sex with men. Subsequent studies indicated that AIDS was also spreading among injection drug users, recipients of blood transfusions, and persons with hemophilia. Then it became apparent that infected pregnant women were transferring the virus to their newborns.

These developments occurred early in the AIDS epidemic. Indeed, even before HIV was isolated, epidemiologists were fairly certain how the virus was spread. Many public health measures and safer sex guidelines have been developed based on their conclusions.

According to the figures from the Centers of Disease Control and Prevention (CDC) discussed in Chapter 4, a total of 711,344 individuals have been identified as AIDS patients in the United States from the beginning of the epidemic in 1981 through 1999. Of this number, 420,201 people have already died. Public health officials estimate that an additional 1 million or more people are infected with HIV and have HIV infection. These individuals are not listed in the current figures, but a notable percentage will likely progress to AIDS. Thus, the AIDS epidemic will continue in the United States into the foreseeable future.

Figure 5.1 shows the statistical breakdown of AIDS cases in the United States from the beginning of the epidemic in 1981 through 1999. The largest percentage occurs in men

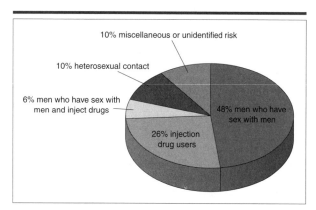

FIGURE 5.1   A summary of the percentage of AIDS cases in various groups since the beginning of the epidemic in 1981.

who have sex with men (48 percent), but the number of cases among injection drug users is also substantial (26 percent). Heterosexual individuals account for 70,582 cases (10 percent). In addition to these figures, the newborns of HIV-infected mothers account for 8596 cases. These distributions have changed over the years, and it is notable that AIDS cases associated with blood transfusions or blood products have declined, primarily because the diagnostic test for HIV helps detect contaminated blood. In addition, modifications of behaviors (discussed in the next chapter) will continue to influence the decrease in the incidence of new HIV infections.

HIV infection is a bloodborne disease known to be transmitted in three major ways: by sexual activity; by transfer of infected blood; and from mother to infant via the placenta or breast milk. There is overwhelming evidence that HIV is not transmitted by casual contact, which implies that family members and healthcare workers will not be infected during the care and treatment of patients. Therefore, most transmission methods are by noncasual methods.

 ## Sexual Transmission

HIV is an extremely fragile virus that rarely survives intact outside the body. Therefore, transmission of HIV almost always requires direct contact between two individuals and depends on a transmission of virus-containing fluid from an infected person to a susceptible person.

For most individuals, the most direct form of contact is sexual contact. Research studies have indicated that, in infected men and women, both semen and vaginal secretions contain HIV. When vaginal intercourse takes place, an infected man deposits HIV-contaminated semen into the cavity of the vagina. Wounds or abrasions in the vaginal mucosa may permit HIV to enter the female's circulatory system in large numbers and establish an infection. Moreover, lesions such as those associated with genital herpes and vaginal warts are associated with a high incidence of HIV transmission because they permit passage of the virus to the deeper tissues. Figure 5.2 depicts these lesions. Furthermore, an underlying sexually transmitted disease such as gonorrhea or chlamydia can hasten transmission because these diseases result in erosion of the tissues lining the reproductive tract and increase the inflammatory response in tissue walls, which increases the likelihood that white blood cells will be present (white blood cells are known to be infection targets of HIV).

During 1997, the CDC investigated an outbreak of HIV infection in upstate rural New York. Forty-seven young women were identified as having had vaginal sex with an HIV-infected male. Of the 47 contacts, 42 were tested, and 13 had HIV infection. These figures represent a 31 percent infection rate, which health officials consider unusually high. Based on the study, public health officials raised the possibility that certain individuals are more efficient transmitters of HIV than

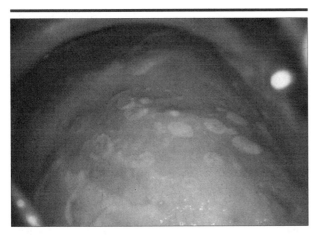

FIGURE 5.2 The lesions of the reproductive organs associated with genital herpes. Lesions such as these facilitate the passage of HIV into the bloodstream and increase the risk of HIV infection.

others, and that these persons may contribute disproportionately to HIV transmission.

Researchers point out that there are reasons for this apparently high transmission rate: persons with primary HIV infection (within several weeks after infection) have unusually high amounts of HIV in the blood, and they can transmit the virus efficiently; and those in the late stages of HIV infection may be particularly infectious, because they have high viral loads. Another possibility is that host susceptibility or the infectiousness of the HIV strain may increase as a result of inflammation or ulceration associated with sexually transmitted disease, as noted previously. The cluster of cases in New York State occurred despite other STD prevention successes in the rural county. The outbreak implies that unrecognized sexual networks of high risk individuals exist, and that public health professionals must provide effective HIV prevention services in rural areas as well as in large cities.

It is now recognized that an HIV-infected woman can transmit HIV to a male. If, for example, HIV is deposited from the vaginal secretions onto the surface of the penis, the foreskin of the penis may hold the infected fluid against the glans, and during this extended period of time, the virus can penetrate through the mucous membranes. Another explanation is that friction occurring during vaginal intercourse may allow viruses to enter through microscopic pores in the wall of the penis.

Among the highest risk behaviors for HIV transmission is anal intercourse. This is because when the penis is inserted into the rectum, there is a high probability of tissue damage and bleeding. The wall of the rectum has a plentiful supply of blood vessels (much water absorption occurs here), and the friction generated during anal intercourse often tears the blood vessels. HIV then passes from semen into the circulation.

Among men who have sex with men, approximately 90 percent of HIV infections are due to the passage of HIV during anal intercourse. The receptive partner is at high risk because HIV is deposited in the rectum, but the insertive partner can also be infected by passage of HIV through the penile wall. Barrier protection can reduce the risk of HIV infection considerably, as discussed in more detail in the next chapter.

It is difficult to assess how many sexual encounters are required for transmission of HIV. For example, some female partners of infected males remain HIV-negative after many months of regular sexual encounters, whereas one or two encounters can result in HIV transmission to other female partners. As we have noted, such factors as underlying diseases, wounds, and abrasions may contribute to the passage of HIV. Conversely, a healthy reproductive system will provide a natural barrier to the passage of HIV.

The number of sexual partners increases the risk of coming in contact with an HIV-infected person. However, this principle is not absolute. For instance, under certain circumstances, sexual encounters with a low number of high risk individuals can be more dangerous than sexual encounters with a large number of low-risk individuals. Also, it should be noted that an individual who has a single sexual partner might be in substantial danger if the partner has had numerous other sexual partners. It has been said that an individual having sex with one person is, in effect, having sex with all the individuals that person has had sex with.

In Africa, the distribution of AIDS cases is more equal among men and women than it is in the United States, where men account for the major number of cases. This equal distribution in Africa indicates to epidemiologists that heterosexual intercourse is the main method for HIV transmission. Female sex workers (prostitutes) are believed to be the major source for HIV in Africa. Residents of major cities and urban areas account for most of the AIDS cases on that continent. For example, public health officials estimate that in certain African cities, as many as 90 percent of female sex workers may be infected.

It should be noted that female-to-female transmission of HIV infection is rare, because sexual activities among lesbians generally do not permit the opportunity for HIV to pass among individuals. In the most unusual circumstances an individual may bleed during sexual contact and permit the virus to gain access to the bloodstream, but these instances have seldom been documented. Health officials advise that latex dental dams be used.

It bears repeating that any sexual activity that produces abrasions prior to or during intercourse may increase the risk of HIV transmission. For example, oral–penile contact is not considered a high risk activity because any HIV ejaculated during oral sex probably normally does not enter the body through the mucosal lining of the mouth. However, the presence of lesions and herpes sores in the mouth raises the risk of transmission, so a latex condom should be used.

Furthermore, intimate kissing is not considered a high risk activity unless numerous lesions are present. The underlying principle is that HIV must have an opportunity to leave the body of the infected individual and enter the bloodstream of the susceptible individual after it has penetrated through the skin barrier.

STDs and AIDS

Since the beginning of the AIDS epidemic, researchers have consistently noted a strong epidemiological association between AIDS and other sexually transmitted diseases (STDs). They have noted the relationship in both developing and industrialized countries, including the United States. The mutual reinforcing nature of these infectious processes has been called "epidemiological synergy." The essential outflow of this synergy is at least a twofold to fivefold increase in the risk for HIV infection among persons who have other STDs. These STDs include ulcerous and inflammatory STDs. Ulcerous STDs include syphilis, chancroid, and herpes simplex virus type 2 (genital herpes). Nonulcerative STDs include gonorrhea, chlamydia (klah-mid'ee-ah), and trichomoniasis (trik-o-mon-i'ah-sis). Bacterial vaginosis (vaj-i-noh'sis) may also increase the risk for HIV infection.

STDs can increase the risk of HIV transmission because ulcers bleed easily and come in contact with the vaginal, cervical, oral, urethral, and rectal mucosa during sexual intercourse. In nonulcerous diseases, inflammation increases the prevalence of HIV shedding and, consequently, increases the amount of HIV in genital secretions. Thus, both types of STDs indicate higher infectiousness of HIV. In one study of note, gonococcal infection in men was shown to increase the shedding of HIV in semen by 10 times; effective treatment of the disease rapidly reduced the HIV shedding to normal levels. In addition, STDs attract T cells to the ulcer surface or cervix, an action that disrupts the mucosal barriers to infection and establishes a possible mechanism to increase susceptibility to HIV infection.

At the present time, the United States has the highest rate of STDs in the industrialized world. In 1998, for example, approximately 600,000 cases of chlamydia were reported to the CDC. (This was the most commonly reported infectious disease in United States, as shown in Figure 5.3.) The incidence of gonorrhea has declined, but in 1998 there were over 355,000 cases, a rate that was 26 times greater than that in Germany. Genital herpes infections are estimated to occur in 45 million persons in the United States in a single year.

It is clear that strategies for reducing STDs will also reduce the incidence of HIV infection and AIDS. This is particularly so when STD prevention is implemented early in an HIV epidemic. Moreover, directing STD interventions toward persons at highest risk for acquiring and transmitting HIV will generate a great impact on the course of an epidemic. Evidence of strategic success is available from studies involving sex workers in countries where HIV transmission was strongly associated with prostitution.

Among the additional steps to enhance STD detection and treatment are those that are designed for early detection and treatment of curable STDs. Improving access to and quality of STD clinical services is also helpful. Public health agencies recommend expanding screening and treatment centers for STDs in medical centers and establishing or expanding screening for STDs in nonmedical centers. For example, all sexually active females under the age of 25 years who visit healthcare providers for any reason should be screened for chlamydia and gonorrhea at least once per year. The same holds true for all young sexually active males. Females can be tested in family-planning clinics, prenatal clinics, emergency rooms, and walk-in clinics as well as community and migrant-worker health centers and school-based clinics. Males also can be tested in walk-in clinics, and many of the other general clinics.

HIV Transmission in Developing Countries

For many years researchers wondered why HIV was being primarily transmitted through heterosexual intercourse in developing countries, when the major routes of infection in industrialized countries have been through the sharing of contaminated needles by injection drug users and by anal intercourse. Researcher Max Essex provided a possible answer when he examined the viruses involved in the HIV epidemic in Thailand and in the United States.

Essex and his research group showed that there is a clear propensity for more efficient infection by the Thailand strain of HIV than by the United States strain. His group learned that HIV from the Thailand strain multiplies rapidly in Langerhans, cells located in the epidermis from the reproductive tract, while the U.S. strain replicates poorly in these cells. Using this evidence, Essex postulated that there are two

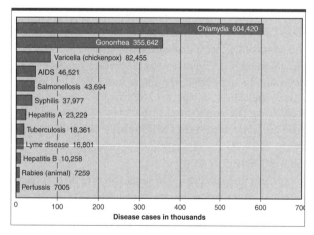

FIGURE 5.3 The reported cases of microbial disease in the United States, 1998. The extremely high prevalence of STDs such as chlamydia, gonorrhea, and syphilis is an important factor in the continuing spread of HIV in the American population.

distinct HIV-1 epidemics. In developed countries, the so-called B subtype predominates and is spread primarily through blood injection and through anal intercourse. By contrast, developing countries experience subtype E HIV; this virus is spread primarily through vaginal intercourse.

Blood to Blood Transmission

Blood to blood transmission of HIV can occur during a blood transfusion or during the transfusion of blood products such as clotting factors required by patients with hemophilia. Early in the AIDS epidemic, these methods were identified as important modes of transmission.

As the epidemic progressed, it became apparent that transmission also is possible via the contaminated instruments employed by injection drug users. It is a common practice among injection drug users to share their "works." When this occurs, the effect is similar to that of a blood transfusion. While injecting drugs, an infected individual inserts a needle into the vein, draws back the plunger to bring blood into the syringe, mixes the blood with the drug, then injects it back into the vein. If the syringe is passed to the next individual without cleaning, any HIV deposited in the syringe will pass to the next person's bloodstream. In the strict sense, blood has been outside the body environment only for a very brief time. Therefore, HIV does not break down, but remains active in the blood. Injection drug users are encouraged not to share their works or related equipment. If this is impossible, then thorough cleaning such as with bleach is recommended. Methods for using disinfectants are surveyed in Chapter 6. Approximately 26 percent of AIDS cases in 1999 were associated with injection drug use, as Table 5.1 demonstrates.

Injection drug users are an important source of HIV passage to the heterosexual population. Users often trade sex for drugs, and sex workers (prostitutes) use sex as a way of obtaining money for support. Indeed, female drug users and the sexual partners of male drug users are a large proportion of the cohort of HIV-infected women. Table 5.1 shows that sex with injection drug users accounted for the highest number of AIDS cases among women from 1998 to 1999. In addition, these women can pass HIV to their newborns.

Blood to blood transmission can also occur among healthcare workers if they sustain punctures with syringes containing contaminated blood ("needlesticks"). Moreover, they can become infected if they contact infected body fluid, as Chapter 7 discusses in more detail. Other individuals who may possibly be exposed to infected blood include emergency medical technicians, dentists, surgeons and physicians, dental hygienists, embalmers and morticians, police officers and firefighters, and correctional facility workers. All should use appropriate cautions for self-protection (Chapter 6).

Blood to blood transmission can also occur from an infected healthcare worker. For example, several years ago a Florida dentist was reported to have presumably transmitted HIV to six patients, although the method for transmission remains unclear. Thus, healthcare workers have an obligation to avoid behaviors that could permit HIV transmission. The risk of obtaining HIV from a healthcare worker, however, is extremely low. Case studies of thousands of patients have revealed relatively few transmissions from an infected healthcare worker.

AIDS in Blood Product Recipients

One of the tragedies of the AIDS epidemics has been the involvement of hemophiliac patients and others who received blood and blood products during transfusions. Hemophiliacs require clotting factors that are obtained from pooled blood. In many cases, 100 pints of blood are used to prepare the clotting factor for a single individual suffering from hemophilia. In the early days of the AIDS epidemic before blood testing was instituted, the risk of HIV-contaminated blood entering into the blood product supply was high, and a great many hemophiliac patients contracted HIV infection and died.

In 1998, the United States Congress approved legislation to compensate hemophiliacs who had contracted HIV during the early years of the epidemic before blood testing was instituted. The legislation gave $100,000 to each of the 7200 hemophiliacs who had contracted HIV through the blood supply or to their surviving family. In addition, legislation provided monetary compensation for 10,000 people infected through blood transfusions such as Ryan White (Figure 5.4).

Mother to Child Transmission

As the AIDS epidemic developed, epidemiologists came to the realization that children can acquire HIV from their mothers by several methods. One method is by perinatal transmission. In this case, the woman's blood is infected with HIV. Although her bloodstream is separated from the child's bloodstream by the placenta, nutrients, small particles, and viruses, can pass across the placental barrier. In this way, HIV can infect the child's bloodstream before it is born.

Another possibility for placental transfer is through small tears in the placenta. Under these circumstances, HIV enters from the mother's bloodstream during the birth process. In addition, when the placenta is disrupted during birth, it is common for the mother's blood to come in contact with the child's blood. In such an instance, HIV transmission can occur.

Public health officials have accumulated evidence indicating that one in two HIV infected women will give birth to an HIV-infected child. This dilemma is a substantial one for a woman who wishes to become pregnant. It should be noted that statistics are approximate and variable. A woman's extent of infection during pregnancy and the duration of infection may be important factors. The CDC classifies all children with AIDS under 13 years of age as "pediatric AIDS cases." Table 5.2

TABLE 5.1 Adult and Adolescent Cases of AIDS Reported to the CDC through June 1999 and Organized by Exposure Category and Gender

	Males				Females				Totals			
	July 1998–June 1999		Cumulative Total		July 1998–June 1999		Cumulative Total		July 1998–June 1999		Cumulative Total	
	No.	(%)	No.	(%)	No.	(%)	No.	(%)	No.	(%)	No.	(%)
Men who have sex with men	15,999	(45)	334,073	(57)	—	—	—	—	15,999	(34)	334,073	(48)
Injection drug use	7,493	(21)	130,727	(22)	3,043	(28)	48,501	(42)	10,536	(23)	179,228	(26)
Men who have sex with men and inject drugs	1,940	(5)	45,266	(8)	—	—	—	—	1,940	(4)	45,266	(6)
Hemophilia/coagulation disorder	150	(0)	4,741	(1)	21	(0)	269	(0)	171	(0)	5,010	(1)
Heterosexual contact:	2,754	(8)	24,984	(4)	4,296	(40)	45,597	(40)	7,051	(15)	70,582	(10)
Sex with injection user	604		8,370		1,208		18,895		1,812		27,265	
Sex with bisexual male	—		—		200		3,263		200		3,263	
Sex with person with hemophilia	7		49		27		396		34		445	
Sex with transfusion recipient with HIV infection	20		382		18		569		38		951	
Sex with HIV-infected person, risk not specified	2,123		16,183		2,843		22,474		4,967		38,658	
Recipient of blood transfusion, blood components, or tissue	146	(0)	4,811	(1)	120	(1)	3,619	(3)	266	(1)	8,430	(1)
Other/risk not reported or identified	7,436	(21)	43,522	(7)	3,361	(31)	16,635	(15)	10,798	(23)	60,159	(9)
Adult/adolescent subtotal	**35,918**	**(100)**	**588,124**	**(100)**	**10,841**	**(100)**	**114,621**	**(100)**	**46,761**	**(100)**	**702,748**	**(100)**

shows the number of pediatric AIDS cases and the probable cause of infection. (The vast majority of the cases are children of color.) Although some cases (4 percent) are a result of blood transfers, the overwhelming number of cases (91 percent) are related to HIV-infected mothers. The fatality rate of such unfortunate children is high. AZT treatment reduces transmission considerably (Chapter 9).

Lack of access to prenatal care or inadequate use of such care is a critical obstacle to maximum reduction of prenatal transmission, especially among women who use illicit drugs. Recent studies have shown that up to 50 percent of women whose HIV infection was detected before they gave birth had no prenatal care. By comparison, in the general population, 4 percent of women giving birth had late or no prenatal care. Women who use illicit drugs during pregnancy are at particularly high risk for not receiving prenatal care because of social disruption, fear of criminal prosecution, and lack of access to care.

Furthermore, there is evidence that HIV can also be transmitted by a nursing mother. During breast-feeding, it is possible that HIV in the breast milk enters the child's body through the gastrointestinal tract by penetrating the tract's lining. The lining consists of mucosa, and in some instances HIV has been known to pass this barrier.

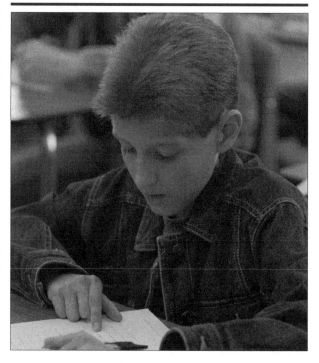

FIGURE 5.4 Ryan White. In the late 1980s, Ryan was barred from school because of an unfounded fear of HIV. His life was later the subject of a television movie.

TABLE 5.2 Pediatric Cases of AIDS Reported to the CDC through June 1999 and Organized by Exposure Category and Gender

	Males				Females				Totals			
	July 1998–June 1999		Cumulative Total		July 1998–June 1999		Cumulative Total		July 1998–June 1999		Cumulative Total	
	No.	(%)	No.	(%)	No.	(%)	No.	(%)	No.	(%)	No.	(%)
Hemophilia/coagulation disorder	1	(1)	226	(5)	—	—	7	(0)	1	(0)	233	(3)
Mother with/at risk for HIV infection:	141	(90)	3,886	(88)	156	(94)	3,942	(95)	297	(92)	7,828	(91)
Injection drug use	38		1,552		37		1,532		75		3,084	
Sex with an injection drug user	27		728		15		691		42		1,419	
Sex with a bisexual male	3		85		1		85		4		170	
Sex with person with hemophilia	—		17		—		12		—		29	
Sex with transfusion recipient with HIV infection	—		11		1		14		1		25	
Sex with HIV-infected person, risk not specified	28		564		45		603		73		1,167	
Recipient of blood transfusion, blood components, or tissue	1		74		1		81		2		155	
Has HIV infection, risk not specified	44		855		56		924		100		1,779	
Recipient of blood transfusion, blood components, or tissue	—	—	236	(5)	—	—	140	(3)	—	—	376	(4)
Risk not reported or identified	14	(9)	80	(2)	10	(6)	79	(2)	24	(7)	159	(2)
Pediatric subtotal	**156**	**(100)**	**4,428**	**(100)**	**166**	**(100)**	**4,168**	**(100)**	**322**	**(100)**	**8,596**	**(100)**

✿ When HIV Is Not Transmitted

It should be clear that HIV passes directly from person to person and is not transmitted casually. Because direct contact is necessary, behaviors and activities that do not involve intimate contact do not transmit HIV. These behaviors and activities are often referred to as casual contact. Therefore, it is safe to say that HIV is not transmitted by casual contact.

Casual contact can imply a number of daily activities of a nonsexual nature. Hugging, kissing, sharing eating utensils are examples of casual contact. Sharing towels, and using the same toilet facilities are additional examples of casual contact. The essential activity in AIDS transmission is the bringing together of body fluids, and casual contact does not imply this. It should also be remembered that HIV breaks down quickly when it is exposed to food, water, or the environment outside the body. Thus, sharing food or swimming in the same environment will not transmit AIDS.

Neither are insects associated with AIDS transmission. If a microorganism is to be transmitted by an insect, it must multiply within the tissues of the insect then make its way to a portal of exit. Malaria parasites, for example, multiply furiously in mosquitoes, then migrate to the salivary glands, and are injected the next time the mosquito bites an individual. No such pattern exists for HIV, and there is no evidence that insects transmit HIV infection.

Finally, it is important to remember that most risky practices can be modified to reduce the possibility of HIV transmission. These modifications are discussed at length in the next chapter.

Questions

1. Explain why unprotected sexual intercourse is a key method for the transmission of HIV and why the presence of a sexually transmitted disease further increases the possibility for transfer.

2. Discuss the circumstances under which HIV is transmitted among injection drug users and from a pregnant woman to her unborn child.

3. Name several methods by which HIV is not transmitted among individuals.

Chapter Six

Preventing HIV Transmission

Review and Preview

We are now well into our study of HIV infection and AIDS. We have seen in previous chapters that AIDS is one of the great challenges confronting the world's health community. We noted in the first chapter that AIDS emerged in American society early in the 1980s, then developed to become a major epidemic of the 20th century that has continued into the 21st century. We also discussed some theories concerning the origin of the human immunodeficiency virus (HIV); we focused on the disease process, and placed HIV into the context of other viruses while examining its structure and pattern of replication. In the early chapters, we saw that HIV wreaks havoc on the helper T cells that modulate the immune system. As the T cell population decreases, the immune defenses of the body are profoundly compromised, and opportunistic illnesses ensue as the person progresses to AIDS. These illnesses can be due to a variety of protozoa, fungi, bacteria, and other microorganisms. The illnesses affect the respiratory, digestive, circulatory, and virtually all other systems of the body. In addition, many AIDS patients suffer dementia and a wasting syndrome.

To deal effectively with the AIDS epidemic, public health epidemiologists study the patterns of the disease in populations and attempt to understand how it is transmitted and spread in the community. In the previous chapter we noted that HIV infection is a bloodborne disease transmitted in three general ways: by sexual activity; by transfer of infected blood by injection drug users; and from mother to infant. Overwhelming evidence indicates that HIV is not transmitted by casual contact.

Because HIV is a fragile virus, it rarely survives intact outside the body, and transmission usually requires direct contact between two individuals and a transmission of fluid from the infected person to the susceptible person. Sexual transmission fulfills these criteria. For example, when semen is deposited in the vagina during vaginal intercourse or in the rectum during anal intercourse, the viruses make their way into the bloodstream of the recipient, especially when wounds, tears, or abrasions in the tissue wall are present. Underlying sexually transmitted diseases such as gonorrhea or syphilis can facilitate the passage of the virus into the bloodstream. It is apparent that a large number of sexual partners increases the risk of coming in contact with an HIV-infected person.

Blood to blood transmission can occur during a blood transfusion or during the transfusion of blood products, such as clotting factors required by patients with hemophilia. Much more commonly, however, injection drug users pass the virus while sharing their needles and syringes. Injection drug users are also an important avenue of HIV infection into the heterosexual population. Although extremely rare, blood to blood transmission can occur if healthcare workers sustain punctures with contaminated syringes or needles.

As the AIDS epidemic developed, it became apparent that newborns can acquire HIV from their mothers by perinatal transmission through the placenta. Exposure to HIV from the mother's bloodstream during the birth process is still another possibility. Moreover, evidence exists that HIV can be transmitted by a woman who nurses her child, because HIV is present in the breast milk.

Knowledge of these methods of transmission is important because health officials can develop and suggest measures to interrupt the transmission of HIV and delay the further spread of the AIDS epidemic. In this chapter we discuss how safer sex practices can interrupt sexual transmission of HIV, how needle disinfection can prevent transmission of HIV among injection drug users, and how counseling and therapy with anti-AIDS medications can limit the possibility of HIV transmission to newborns. Furthermore, it may be possible for the HIV-infected patient to delay the progression to AIDS by avoiding the opportunistic illnesses that signal AIDS. For example, avoiding such animals as cats can reduce the risk for acquiring toxoplasmosis. Finally, we will see how the blood supply can be made safe so that individuals can avoid HIV infection during blood transfusions. While the scientific community continues to search out and develop new therapies and vaccines, prevention is a primary method for dealing with the AIDS epidemic.

Introduction

More than two decades after it was first described, the AIDS pandemic continues in the United States and around the world. The Centers for Disease Control and Prevention (CDC) estimates that over a million persons are infected annually with HIV in the United States. In the absence of a curative treatment or a vaccine, prevention of HIV transmission becomes essential for controlling the epidemic.

Epidemiological and ethnographic studies indicate that most cases of HIV transmission are linked to some type of human behavior (Chapter 5), and thus, transmission can be interrupted by changing the behavior. For example, researchers have discovered that needle exchange programs can reduce the incidence of AIDS among populations who use injection drugs and habitually share contaminated needles.

The research has also made it clear that the effectiveness of a prevention program is inexorably linked to how consistently the program is applied to behavioral changes. Inadequate patient education, lack of access to drug treatment programs, and inconsistent application of risk reduction programs encourage individuals to revert to previous behaviors, rendering the behavioral change program ineffective.

The methods for preventing HIV transmission are linked to the methods through which the virus is known to move from individual to individual. Some methods focus on preventing person to person transmission, while other methods concentrate on decontaminating drug paraphernalia, and still others stress counseling and patient education.

Safer Sex Practices

Two decades of intense study have led researchers to the conclusion that HIV infection is not highly contagious. Among the major modes of transmission of HIV is sexual transmission because sexual contact affords a fragile virus such as HIV an opportunity to move directly from individual to individual, tissue to tissue, cell to cell.

Paramount to preventing transmission is a change in social behavior. Sexual abstinence remains the principal method for interrupting the sexual transmission of HIV, but a mutually monogamous sexual relationship can be equally important because it severely limits the opportunities to encounter HIV. Appropriate barrier protection used during sexual activity (i.e., latex condoms) can effectively diminish the possibility of transmitting HIV as well. Abstinence and a mutually monogamous relationship are endorsed by the Surgeon General of the United States as the preferred methods for preventing HIV transmission. Barrier prevention methods are the next preferred method.

To prevent the transmission of sexually transmitted diseases such as AIDS, individuals should use condoms, diaphragms, and/or latex dams all of which contain spermicide. (Spermicides are commercially available as creams, foams, and jellies, and in suppositories and sponges.) A condom used with a spermicide is the recommended barrier protection against HIV, and quality control guidelines enforced by the U.S. Food and Drug Administration ensure protection against defects. Condoms provide a physical barrier between ejaculated semen and lesions present in the vagina, anus, or oral cavity. Unfortunately, some materials used to make condoms can cause an allergic skin reaction, known as contact dermatitis. For example, the latex in latex condoms is allergenic to a small percentage of individuals in the United States.

Most health officials recommend using condoms having the spermicide called nonoxynol-9 (no-nox'i-nil-9). Unfortunately, this drug is a nonspecific inhibitor of microorganisms, that is, in addition to eliminating HIV, herpesvirus, and other harmful organisms, the drug also eliminates helpful bacteria such as lactobacilli, which are commonly found in the woman's vagina. These bacteria maintain the acidity of this organ, thereby preventing other organisms from infecting it. When the lactobacilli are killed by the drug, the acidity disappears, and other microorganisms invade the urinary tract. (Often they arrive from the opening to the anus, which is near the vaginal opening.) The bacteria invade through the urethra and invade the woman's bladder, where they cause urinary tract infections. In view of this finding, women with a history of urinary tract infections should avoid contraceptives having nonoxynol-9.

The risk of HIV transmission varies with the type of sexual practices in which individuals engage. Among the most dangerous sexual practices are vaginal intercourse without a condom, and anal intercourse without a condom. Body fluids containing potentially high concentrations of HIV may be transmitted during these times, and direct contact with target sites is possible. Extensive epidemiological evidence documents the strong relationship between sexual intercourse and HIV infection. A condom should be placed on the erect penis prior to penetration, and it should be used with a water-based lubricant, rather than a grease-based or oil-based lubricant, both of which can weaken the latex. The condom should remain in place until the penis is withdrawn from the vagina or anus.

Among the less hazardous but still risky sexual practices are oral sex on a man if a condom is not used, and oral sex on a woman. The exchange of potentially contaminated body fluids could occur, and there is potential for contact with lesions in the mouth and throat. Should this contact be made, HIV can be transmitted into the bloodstream.

In the next group of less risky practices is vaginal intercourse using a condom, anal intercourse using a condom, and passionate kissing. Condom use lessens the possibility for passage of body fluids, while open-mouth passionate kissing poses a possible risk because of the extensive contact with potentially contaminated saliva. The concentration of HIV found in saliva is extremely low; hence the risk from passionate kissing is also low.

Among the safer sexual practices are touching, dry kissing, and masturbation. These practices and others are considered "safer" because contact with susceptible cells is not made. Although contaminated semen might be present, the risk remains low.

Healthcare providers have an important place in preventing the transmission of HIV. Physicians should incorporate discussions of sexuality and drug use into their clinical practices. Furthermore, a physician may engage a patient in a structured discussion of safer sexual practices, depending on the availability of adequate time and privacy. The physician may reinforce the importance of condom use and a mutually monogamous relationship, while highlighting the patient's personal investment in the behavioral change. Furthermore, the physician should support the patient's efforts to discuss high risk behaviors with sexual partners. Sexual histories can be reviewed to assist further in evaluating the risk for HIV infection. Topics should be tailored to the patient's lifestyle and risk behaviors, and the goal for risk reduction should be to create an impetus for behavioral change involving self-care as well as protection of others.

 ## Safer Injection Drug Use Practices

In CDC statistics compiled through mid-1999, injection drug users accounted for 26 percent of diagnosed cases of AIDS in adults and adolescents. Accordingly, injection drug users constitute the second largest transmission group, after men who have sex with men (48 percent). Indeed, sexual contact with injection drug users often accounts for the spread of HIV to the heterosexual population—through the end of the 1990s, half of the women who harbored HIV were infected through injection drug use and almost one-quarter were infected through heterosexual contact with an injection drug user. Over one-half of pediatric cases of AIDS occur in children of injection drug users or their sexual partners.

The term injection drug user has replaced the term intravenous drug user because researchers have discovered that injections can be made in a number of ways other than intravenously. For example, intramuscular (in the muscle) or subcutaneous (under the skin) injection of drugs is possible. Thus, "injection drug user" a more inclusive term, has been adopted. Although injection drug users can belong to any of these groups, intravenous injection of drugs remains the most important method for HIV transmission among drug users. In addition to elicit street drugs such as heroin, steroids and amphetamines are also injected.

In most cases, needle sharing accounts for cross-infection among drug users as described in Chapter 5. Following injection, the needle and the syringe both retain some of the user's blood, and if the apparatus is used directly by the next individual, the contaminated blood is also transmitted. And because injection drugs sometimes compromise the immune system, HIV infection can occur at an accelerated pace. In addition, contaminated blood can transmit other diseases such as hepatitis B and hepatitis C. However, studies indicate that the time of progression from HIV infection to AIDS is similar in injection drug users and other infected populations.

Several important issues confront women. For example, women may contract HIV from sexual partners who have become infected by others. Furthermore, a woman may give birth to a baby who is infected with HIV or addicted to drugs, or both. Psychological issues are involved because women develop a poor self-image. Moreover, women who support themselves by exchanging sex for drugs or money constitute another population with unique needs and a unique outlook. Women should be counseled about the possibilities of giving birth to an HIV-infected infant or about the loss of custody because of their sickness or drug use. Thus, explaining the medical, psychological, and social issues to HIV-infected women who are injection drug users requires understanding their unique perspective.

Drug treatment of injection drug users who are HIV-positive may be difficult because drug users seek medical services only when in crisis. There is also the issue of noncompliance with appointments and treatment regimens. Furthermore, healthcare providers may be concerned about their own health when treating injection drug users, especially as a disproportionate number of drug users have tuberculosis, which is spread by airborne droplets of mucus and saliva. In addition, injection drug users are frequently treated with disrespect because they are viewed as self-destructive, antisocial, and violent. They often lack health insurance, which makes treatment and interrupting HIV transmission among members of this group particularly difficult.

Outreach workers have been trained to provide information to injection drug users in their environment. These workers are often of the same community, ethnic background, and race as the drug users and they can often relate to their plight because they may be recovered drug users themselves. Because injection drug users have long histories of drug use, advising them to simply quit is not an effective method. Rather, the better alternative is to advise them on the safe use of sterile needles, syringes, and other injection equipment. Instruction should be given about methods for cleaning needles, syringes, and other paraphernalia.

The CDC recommends a 10 percent dilution of household bleach as an effective cleansing agent. This is prepared by adding one teaspoon of bleach to nine teaspoons of water. (More concentrated or full strength bleach may be used if it is not feasible to prepare 10 percent bleach.) Before using the bleach, the needle and syringe should be washed out several times with clean water. The syringe should then be placed in the bleach and drawn up and released several times, with several rinses. The bleach should be allowed to remain in the syringe for a few seconds or up to one minute. Rinses in water should then follow. (The water used for rinsing the syringe should be fresh each time.) The syringe should be filled completely to the top and it should be tapped or shaken while being filled to improve the effectiveness of the washing. The syringe should be taken apart and placed in the cup of bleach where possible.

Unfortunately, clotted blood is more difficult to remove than fresh blood, and the bleach method is not completely effective. HIV inactivation is not certain in this situation, but consistent and thorough cleaning of injection equipment reduces the possibility of HIV transmission considerably.

Carrying a bottle of bleach at all times can be hazardous, but public health officials suggest it may be an effective way of having materials available for cleaning the syringe. The cap of the container should have a foil insert to prevent the bleach from contacting and weakening the cap. Local laws and regulations affect needle and syringe availability and possession, but even in states where carrying drug paraphernalia is illegal, a bleach bottle does not constitute drug paraphernalia.

Syringe Exchange Programs

Because so many cases of AIDS are associated with injection drug use, syringe exchange programs are a key strategy in preventing infection with HIV (Figure 6.1). The goal of syringe exchange programs is to reduce transmission of HIV and other bloodborne infections by providing sterile syringes in exchange for used and potentially contaminated syringes. In this discussion, the term syringe refers to both the syringe and its needle.

Survey results indicate continuing growth in the number, geographic coverage, and activity of syringe exchange programs in the United States. From 1995 to 1997, for example, health officials reported a 74 percent increase in the number of programs in participating cities. (A total of 80 cities were participating as of 1997.) The number of syringes exchanged rose from 8 million in 1995 to 17.5 million in 1997. Programs received financial support from various sources, including foundations, individuals, and state and local governments. It should be noted, however, that current federal law prohibits the use of federal funds to carry out an exchange program for materials involving the hypodermic injection of any illegal drug.

Locations for syringe exchange programs include home visits, storefront locations, vans, sidewalk tables, health clinics, and locations where injection drug users gather to inject drugs ("shooting galleries"). The programs often include community outreach programs, HIV-prevention programs in jails and prisons, counseling against initiating drug use, and health care for HIV-infected drug users. In many U.S. states the program is allowed to operate by law. Other services pro-

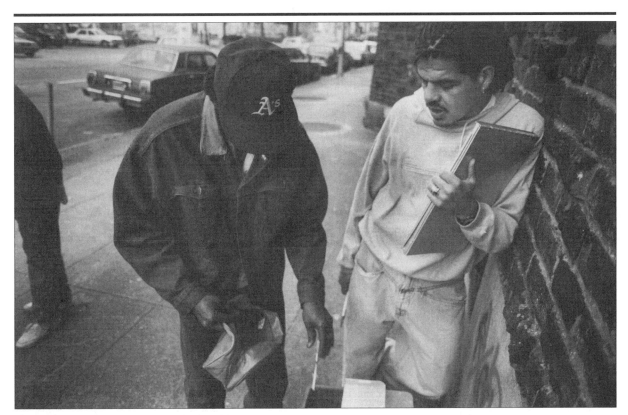

FIGURE 6.1 Syringe exchange programs effectively reduce the incidence of HIV infection among injection drug users. Each year, over 20 million contaminated syringes are exchanged for sterile ones in such programs.

vided by the centers include client referrals to substance abuse clinics, STD prevention education, and instruction in the use of condoms and dental dams to prevent sexual transmission of HIV infection and other sexually transmitted diseases. Also included are HIV counseling and testing, tuberculosis skin testing, and STD screenings.

Syringe exchange centers are not allowed to operate in states having laws restricting the purchase of hypodermic needles or in states providing exemption to the prescription-only laws. Despite the increasing numbers of people taking advantage of syringe exchange programs, the actual number of injection drug users has not increased but rather has stabilized over the last few years, according to CDC statistics. Among the surprises of the program are the numbers of syringe exchanges taking place in traditionally conservative areas not known for their drug problems. Communities that in the past would not acknowledge a drug problem are realizing that the programs help the community in numerous ways. The downside is that, with the increasing number and efficiency of the programs, the numbers of syringes exchanged also increase and additional monies are needed to support the programs.

 ## Safety for Healthcare Workers

Occupational transmission of HIV among healthcare workers has been a cause of concern since the beginning of the AIDS epidemic. However, several studies have shown that the risk of infection following occupational exposure to HIV-infected blood or body fluids is quite low, usually less than 1 percent. This figure implies that since the beginning of the AIDS epidemic, less than 1 percent of those exposed during their workday developed HIV infection or AIDS as a result of contact with blood or body fluid. Chapter 7 explores HIV and healthcare workers in depth. Because safety precautions to minimize risk are surveyed in that chapter, we will not cover them here.

 ## Prenatal AIDS Counseling

Beginning in July 1995, the U.S. Public Health Service recommended that healthcare providers counsel pregnant women about HIV prevention and encourage them to be tested for HIV infection. If the tests were positive, health officials recommended therapy with azidothymidine (AZT), also known as zidovudine (ZDV). This program was entitled the Pregnancy Risk Assessment Monitoring System.

When researchers assessed the program some years later, they found that a substantial number of women had undergone HIV tests. In 1997, over 70% of women in nine states recalled discussing HIV testing with their healthcare provider during prenatal care, and at least 50 percent of women all states reported being tested for HIV during pregnancy or at delivery. Not surprisingly, in states with high HIV infection rates,

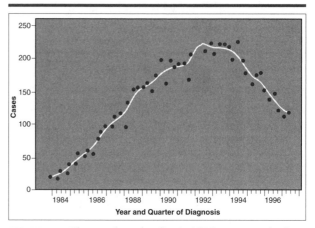

FIGURE 6.2   The number of pediatric AIDS cases acquired perinatally over a multiyear period. The dropoff in cases beginning in the 1992 time period coincides with the first use of AZT therapy in pregnant women.

healthcare providers placed a higher priority on prenatal HIV prevention than in states with low infection rates. Differences in state laws also contributed to variations in HIV discussions and testing. During 1996, for example, the states of Florida and New York enacted legislation requiring that all healthcare providers include HIV counseling during prenatal care.

The risk of HIV transmission from mother to infant has been considerably reduced by the use of antiretroviral therapy, as shown in Figure 6.2. However, in developing countries anti-HIV drugs are very expensive. Moreover, improvement is needed identifying women with HIV-infection before pregnancy or early in pregnancy so that they and their infants can be offered the full benefit of therapy. Also, new antiretroviral agents need to be researched as alternatives for use in patients where the AZT causes side effects. Research is also needed on the use of anti-HIV antibodies (gamma globulin) to neutralize HIV in the bloodstream.

 ## Avoiding Opportunistic Pathogens

To avoid transmission of opportunistic pathogens during sexual exposures, individuals at risk should use a latex condom during each act of sexual intercourse. This will reduce the risk for acquiring of HIV as well as cytomegalovirus (si-to-meg'a-lo-vi-rus, also called CMV), herpes simplex virus, and human papillomavirus (pap-i-lo'-mah-vi-rus), as well as other sexually transmitted pathogens.

Condom use may also reduce the risk of acquiring human herpesvirus 8, which is related to Kaposi's sarcoma, as well as a second infection (a superinfection) with a strain of HIV resistant to antiretroviral drugs. In addition, patients should avoid sexual practices that might result in exposure to feces to reduce the risk of intestinal infection such as cryptosporidiosis (krip"-to-spor-id-i-o'sis), hepatitis A, and campylobacteriosis (kam"-pi-lo-bac-ter-i-o'sis), an intestinal disease accompanied by severe diarrhea.

For individuals who are injection drug users, exposure to opportunistic pathogens can be reduced as well. Injection drug use puts HIV-infected persons at risk for hepatitis B virus infection, plus infection with strains of various bacteria and other blood borne pathogens. Patients should be counseled to stop using injection drugs and enter a substance-abuse program.

If they continue to inject drugs, patients should be advised to never reuse or share syringes, needles, or drug preparation equipment. If they do share, they should first clean the equipment with bleach and water, as noted earlier. They should be advised to use sterile syringes obtained from reliable sources such as pharmacies or syringe exchange programs. Moreover, they should be counseled to use boiled water to prepare drugs or, if impossible, to use clean water from a reliable source. A disinfected container and a new filter should be used to prepare their drugs. Cleaning the injection site with an alcohol swab before injection is helpful as well.

To decrease their risk of exposure to tuberculosis, HIV-infected individuals should consider discontinuing such activities as volunteer work or employment in healthcare facilities, correctional institutions, shelters for homeless, and other settings identified as high risk environments by local health authorities. Decisions should be based on such factors as patient's specific duties in a workplace, the prevalence of tuberculosis in the community, and the degree to which precautions for preventing tuberculosis transmission are taken in the workplace.

Childcare providers and parents of children in childcare facilities are at risk for acquiring CMV infection, cryptosporidiosis, and other infection such as hepatitis A from children. The risk can be diminished by good hygienic practices, such as handwashing after changing diapers and after contact with urine.

Avoiding Animalborne Pathogens

Occupations involving animal contact such as veterinary work and employment in pet stores or slaughterhouses might pose a risk for acquiring the pathogens that cause diseases affecting both humans and animals. These include toxoplasmosis (tok'-soh-plaz-moh'sis), salmonellosis, campylobacteriosis, or *Bartonella* infection (cat scratch fever), as well as cryptosporidiosis. Therefore, adequate precautions should be taken to avoid contact with contaminated items. In addition, contact with the young farm animals, especially those with diarrhea should be avoided to reduce the risk of acquiring cryptosporidiosis caused by *Cryptosporidium* (Figure 6.3).

Handwashing after gardening or other contact with the soil is another useful way of reducing possible exposure to opportunistic pathogens. For those living in areas endemic for histoplasmosis (his'-to-plaz-mo'sis), patients should avoid creating dust when working with soil, cleaning chicken coops

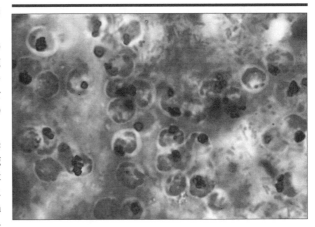

FIGURE 6.3 An electron micrograph of *Cryptosporidium*, the protozoal parasite that causes cryptosporidiosis. This parasite causes a severe and unrelenting diarrhea in AIDS patients. It can be avoided by reducing association with farm animals and not drinking water from rivers and streams.

contaminated with droppings, disturbing the soil beneath bird-roosting sites, cleaning old buildings, and exploring caves. In addition, where there is possibility for coccidioidomycosis (kok"-sid-i-oi'do-mi-ko-sis), patients should avoid dust from exposure to local soil, because the responsible fungi exist here.

To avoid opportunistic pathogens obtained from pets, certain precautions are also worth considering. (However, counselors should be sensitive to the psychological benefits of pet ownership and should advise HIV-infected patients to part with their pets only as a last resort.) When a pet develops diarrheal illness, HIV-infected individuals should avoid contact with the animal and have it examined by a competent veterinarian. When obtaining a new pet, they should avoid animals aged less than 6 months (or less than 1 year for cats), especially if the animal has diarrhea. Hygienic and sanitary conditions in animal shelters tend to be highly variable, so the patient should be cautious when obtaining a pet from these sources. Stray animals should be avoided. Patients should wash their hands after handling pets, especially before eating, and should avoid contact with the pet's feces.

With respect to cats, patients should be advised that owning cats increases their risk for toxoplasmosis and *Bartonella* infection. Litterboxes should be cleaned daily, preferably by an HIV-negative individual who is not pregnant. (The pregnancy precaution is because toxoplasmosis can infect a pregnant woman, and the responsible microbe can pass across the placental barrier to her unborn child.) If the HIV-infected individual must perform this task, the hands should be washed thoroughly.

Patients should keep their cats indoors, and prevent them from hunting. Cats should not be fed raw or under-cooked meat (as *Toxoplasma* is often found here). HIV-infected individuals should avoid any activities that might result in scratches from a cat. This will reduce the risk for *Bartonella* infection, which leads to cat scratch disease. Cats should not be allowed to lick a patient's open wounds or cuts. Flea control to reduce the risk for *Bartonella* infection in the cat is advisable.

Other pets also transmit opportunistic pathogens, so caution is advised. Contact with reptiles, for example, should be avoided to reduce the risk for salmonellosis. Snakes, lizards, turtles, and iguanas are all included in this list. When cleaning aquariums, gloves should be worn to reduce the risk of contact with *Mycobacterium marinum*, a marine bacterium that can cause lung disease.

Avoiding Foodborne and Waterborne Pathogens

Food and water may also be sources of opportunistic pathogens, and HIV-infected individuals must take precautions. Raw or undercooked eggs or foods may be a source of the *Salmonella* species that cause intestinal illness. Raw or undercooked poultry and meat, and unpasteurized dairy products may also contain intestinal pathogens. Poultry and meat should be cooked until no longer pink in the middle, and they should reach an internal temperature higher than 165°F. Produce should be thoroughly washed before being eaten.

To avoid contact with *Cryptosporidium* and *Giardia*, HIV-infected individuals should not drink water directly from lakes or rivers. Water swallowed during recreational activities might also be a source of these pathogens, so caution should be taken while swimming. If a "boil water advisory" is issued in the community, water should be boiled for one minute to eliminate the risk for acquiring cryptosporidiosis. Using personal-use water filters and drinking bottled water reduce the risk further. Ice from contaminated water may also be a source of infection. Fountain beverages and drinks in restaurants, bars, and theaters might pose a risk when the beverages contain ice made from local water.

Travel, particularly to developing countries, might pose a health risk for an HIV-infected person. Raw fruits and vegetables, raw or undercooked seafood or meat, unpasteurized milk and dairy products, and items purchased from street vendors might be contaminated and be a source of opportunistic pathogens. Steaming-hot foods, fruits peeled by the traveler, bottled beverages, hot coffee, beer, wine, and boiled water are generally safe to consume.

Many physicians consider antimicrobial pretreatments and preventatives for diarrhea to be of limited value for travelers because the drugs have adverse effects on the body and promote the emergence of drug-resistant microbes. However, when doctors do recommend prophylaxis to reduce the risk for diarrhea among travelers, the fluoroquinolone (floor-o-quin'o-lone) antibiotics such as ciprofloxacin (sip-ro-flox'a-sin) can be considered. In addition, counselors should advise HIV-infected individuals about other preventative travel

measures. This might include prophylaxis for malaria, treatment with immune globulin, and various vaccines. It is well to remember that many tropical and developing areas have high rates of tuberculosis, and travelers should be advised about area-specific risks.

Safety of the Blood Supply

During 1985, the United States Public Health Service implemented testing for HIV antibodies in all blood donated by individuals. The first tests were designed to detect HIV-1. Testing resulted in a substantial decrease in transmission of HIV through blood transfusions. In 1992, the testing of all blood for HIV-2 as well as HIV-1 was implemented. A combination antibody test was used.

The risk for HIV transmission through transfusion of screened blood is now minimal. Nearly all cases of transfusion-associated HIV transmission are a result of blood that was donated during the period when a recently infected donor possessed the virus but had not yet developed detectable levels of HIV antibody. During the years between 1985 and 1990, enzyme immunosorbent assays (Chapter 8) were used to screen blood, and the average length of the "window period" between infection and the appearance of antibodies was 45 days. Since that time, assays have been produced with more sensitivity, and the average infectious window period is about 25 days. A further improvement noted below can improve the window period to about 16 days.

In addition, improved donor interviewing has also helped improve blood safety. The safety has been even further improved by deferring donors who test positive for hepatitis or syphilis. In 1993, approximately 6 per 100,000 blood donations collected by the U.S. Red Cross tested positive for HIV antibodies. Moreover, an estimated 1 in 450,000 to 1 in 660,000 donations per year (18 to 27 donations) were infectious for HIV but were not detected by the improved screening tests now in use.

The safety of the blood supply can further be improved by testing for the p24 antigen of HIV, because this antigen can be detected earlier than antibodies. The p24 antigen is at the core protein of HIV. It is detectable two to three weeks after HIV has entered the body and during the initial burst of virus replication, a period associated with high levels of viremia. On average, the p24 antigen is detected about six days before antibody tests become positive. Once the antibodies are detectable, the p24 antigen appears to disappear from the blood, probably because of its reaction with HIV antibodies.

Beginning in August 1995, the U.S. Food and Drug Administration recommended that all blood and plasma donations be screened for p24 antigen. Among the 12 million pints of blood annually donated in the United States, the p24 antigen test detects four to six cases when the blood is infectious with HIV. Other screening tests would not identify HIV at such an early stage. As of 2000, the chance that a pint of blood used for transfusion will be contaminated with HIV is 1 in 676,000.

To lower the window period still farther, blood collection facilities including the American Red Cross are beginning to implement nucleic acid amplification testing. Instead of detecting viral antibodies or p24 antigen, the test zeros in on a genetic material of the virus itself. The test uses the polymerase chain reaction (PCR) to amplify ("copy") viral RNA particles millions of times. Then the particles can be detected. This technique makes it possible to locate as few as 100 viral particles per milliliter of blood. Using this test, HIV may be detectable as soon as ten days after infection.

Applying the test to each donated pint of blood would probably be impractical. Therefore, blood centers are using a pooling method. In this procedure, they take samples from donations and pool them together to test them all at one time. The sensitivity of the testing remains, but the cost is substantially reduced. A typical master pool contains 128 samples. If the master pool tests positive then each of the primary pools are tested. Eight smaller primary pools make up the master pool and each of the eight primary pools contains 16 samples. If the primary pool tests positive then the additional samples of 16 are then tested. As of mid-1999, over 50 percent of all donated blood was being tested by this method. Testing and the other safety precautions discussed in this chapter help to ensure that AIDS does not extend its established boundaries.

Questions

1. Which safer sex practices can be used to help prevent the spread of HIV?

2. Discuss the recommendations for injection drug users to interrupt the transmission of HIV among individuals.

3. What measures can be taken to avoid the opportunistic pathogens associated with AIDS?

Chapter Seven

AIDS and Healthcare Workers

Review and Preview

As we enter the 21st century, the AIDS epidemic continues in the United States and around the world. According to estimates by the CDC, over 1 million persons are infected with HIV in the United States and over 30 million individuals harbor the virus in the global community. The virus attacks the helper T cells of the immune system and destroys them, thereby subjecting the body to a variety of opportunistic illnesses and cancers. A wasting syndrome and brain-centered dementia are other characteristics found in certain AIDS patients. In the absence of a curative treatment or vaccine, prevention of HIV transmission is essential to controlling the epidemic.

In the previous chapters, we learned how HIV infects cells of the body and how HIV spreads among individuals in the community. By understanding the mode of transmission, public health agencies can work to interrupt the transmission. For example, health officials recommend safer sex practices to prevent the transmission of virus via the sexual mode. They provide evidence that barrier protection such as latex condoms can effectively prevent HIV transmission during sexual activity.

Fully one-quarter of all diagnosed cases of AIDS in adults are associated with injection drug users. Following injection of drugs, the needle and syringe retains some of the user's blood, and if the apparatus is passed directly to the next individual, contaminated blood is also transmitted. Therefore, it is important to use clean, sterile needles and when this is not possible, to clean the needle and syringe with disinfectants such as bleach. Needle exchange programs have been shown to be effective ways of discouraging the spread of HIV, and at this writing, many of the U.S. states have such programs in operation.

Because HIV passes across the placenta to the unborn fetus, healthcare providers have begun counseling programs to inform pregnant women about AIDS and encourage them to be tested for HIV infection. If they test positive, treatment with azidothymidine can substantially reduce the possibility of HIV passage to the newborn.

For those who are already infected, it may be possible to delay the progression to AIDS by avoiding the pathogens that cause opportunistic illnesses. For example, avoiding exposure to animals can reduce the possibility of coming in contact with such pathogens as *Cryptosporidium, Toxoplasma, Salmonella,* and *Bartonella.* Handwashing after gardening is another way of reducing exposure to soilborne pathogens. And travel to developing countries can be limited as a way of reducing exposure to other pathogens.

One group of individuals that has been at risk since AIDS surfaced is the corps of healthcare workers. Despite working regularly with HIV-infected patients, members of this group have developed relatively few infections, which probably attests to their professionalism and caution while helping patients. The low number of transmissions also points up the fact that HIV is not easily transmitted among individuals, while reinforcing the effectiveness of practices universally in place in healthcare settings as part of infection control programs.

Nevertheless, some risk does exist for healthcare workers, and this chapter examines some of those risks. We will outline how transmission of HIV can take place, and examine some of the universal precautions now encouraged to prevent that transmission. Transmission is sometimes a fact of life, but therapies are available to healthcare workers to forestall the progression to AIDS. Because healthcare workers stand on the front lines of the healthcare system, we pay them special attention and devote a chapter to their special needs.

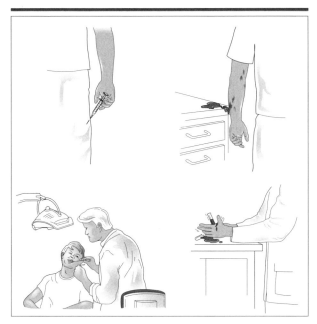

FIGURE 7.1 Four possible modes for transfer of HIV to healthcare workers.

Introduction

One of the primary considerations during the course of the AIDS epidemic has been the safety of the professional who cares for the health of AIDS patients. The healthcare worker is one whose activity involves contact with patients or with blood or other body fluids from patients in a healthcare or laboratory setting. Such a person may be an employee, a student, an attending clinician, or a public safety worker.

For healthcare workers, precautions should be in place to prevent injuries caused by needles, scalpel blades, and other sharp instruments or devices. Because HIV does not survive well outside the body, the virus can be destroyed with relative ease, and healthcare workers should always follow good handwashing techniques, particularly if hands are contaminated with blood or other body fluids. Commonly used germicides rapidly inactivate HIV and should be used regularly. Indeed, standard sterilization and disinfection procedures are generally adequate to destroy HIV.

Having noted some of these general insights, we now study some specifics of how AIDS affects healthcare workers. We shall begin with the modes of HIV transmission to these individuals.

✳ Transmission of HIV Among Healthcare Workers

Exposure to HIV in the workplace may occur by any of a number of means, including percutaneous injury such as a cut with a sharp object or a needlestick. Exposure may also occur as a result of blood or body fluid contact with the mucous membrane or damaged skin of the worker. This is a mucocutaneous exposure, as shown in Figure 7.1. The skin can be damaged when it is abraded, chapped, or has dermatitis.

An exposure can also occur between intact skin and virus-containing material when the duration of contact with body fluid is several minutes or more, or when it involves an extensive area of skin. Contact involves body fluids such as semen, casual secretions, or other body fluids contaminated with visible blood that have been implicated in HIV transmission. The contact can also involve cerebrospinal, synovial, pleural, peritoneal, pericardial, or amniotic fluids. The risk of these latter fluids transmitting HIV has not been determined. In addition, any direct contact with concentrated HIV in a research laboratory or an industrial facility is considered an exposure when barrier protection was not used. This exposure requires clinical evaluation and a possible need for preventive treatment following the exposure. Such treatment is known as postexposure prophylaxis.

At the time of this writing, only one nonoccupational episode of HIV transmission has been attributed to contact with blood-contaminated saliva. This incident involved intimate kissing between sexual partners. Such contact is not similar to contact with saliva that may occur while healthcare services are being provided. Therefore, when blood is absent in the saliva, exposure to saliva from an individual infected with HIV is not considered a risk factor for HIV transmission. Health officials point out that exposure to tears, sweat, or urine free of blood or feces does not to require postexposure prophylaxis.

Human breast milk has been implicated in perinatal transmission of HIV. However, healthcare workers exposed to human breast milk have not acquired HIV. Indeed, the contact that a healthcare worker may have had with human breast milk is considerably different from the perinatal exposure that an infant has with an HIV-infected mother.

The possibility of HIV transmission through soiled laundry and soiled linen is not considered high. Common sense storage and normal hygiene and processing are recommended, although soiled linen should be handled as little as possible and with minimum agitation to prevent microbial contamination of the air. Hospital wastes requiring special precautions include microbiology laboratory waste, pathology waste, blood specimens, and blood products. It should be noted that the patient with HIV infection does not require isolation because of the presence of HIV. However, isolation may be required because of any opportunistic illnesses the patient has. For example, lung infection with *Pneumocystis carinii* may necessitate isolation because this organism can be passed in droplets of mucus expelled during coughing.

Risk of HIV Transmission

Studies of healthcare workers have estimated that the average risk for HIV transmission after a percutaneous exposure to HIV-contaminated blood is approximately 0.3 percent (within

95 percent confidence limits). After a mucous membrane exposure, the average risk for HIV transmission is 0.09 percent. The risk for transmission after skin exposure is estimated to be less than the risk for mucous membrane exposure.

As of June 1999, the U.S. Centers for Disease Control and Prevention (CDC) had received reports of 55 healthcare workers in the United States having contracted HIV infection after exposure to HIV. An additional 136 episodes in healthcare workers are considered "possible" occupational transmissions of HIV; the workers in these episodes reported that they had no other risk for HIV infection (e.g., injection drug use), but transmission of infection after the exposure could not be fully documented. In the 55 documented episodes cited above, 50 healthcare workers were exposed to infected blood, one was exposed to body fluids having visible blood, three were exposed to concentrated virus in a laboratory, and one to an unspecified fluid. Forty-seven exposures were percutaneous, and five were mucocutaneous. Two healthcare workers had both percutaneous and mucocutaneous exposures. Of the percutaneous exposures, hollow-bore needles were involved in the majority of cases, a broken glass file was involved in two cases, a scalpel in one case, and an unknown sharp object in a final case. Twenty-five of the 55 individuals progressed to AIDS as of the date of the report (Table 7.1).

Several factors may affect the risk for HIV transmission. For an occupational exposure, the risk for HIV transmission increases with exposure to a large quantity of blood from the source patient. The risk also increases if exposure has taken place with blood from a patient having terminal illness. The latter probably reflects the high amount of HIV in the blood late in the course of the disease. Furthermore, there is evidence that host defense may influence the possibility for HIV infection because a healthy host may develop a vigorous immune response to prevent establishment of HIV infection following exposure. The universal precautions discussed next help to lower the possibility of transmission.

 ## Universal Precautions

Although the possibility of HIV transmission from patients to healthcare workers is relatively low, a major effort has been made by public health agencies to reduce the likelihood of such transmission. The principles underlying this effort are called universal precautions. They should be followed when caring for all patients, including those known to be positive for HIV. This is important because even though laboratory tests may fail to identify HIV antibodies, the person may be infected with HIV.

The universal precautions dictate that all healthcare workers should routinely use appropriate barrier precautions to prevent skin and mucous membrane exposure during contact with blood or other body fluids of a patient. Gloves should be worn for touching body and body fluids, mucous membranes, or nonintact skin of all patients; for handling items or surfaces soiled with blood or body fluids; and for performing venipuncture and other vascular access procedures. Gloves should be changed after contact with each patient.

Masks and protective eyewear or face shields should be worn during procedures that will likely generate droplets of blood or other body fluids. The protection will prevent expo-

TABLE 7.1 Cases of HIV Infection in Healthcare Workers Acquired During the Course of Their Work Through 1999.

Occupation	Documented Occupational Transmission	Possible Occupational Transmission
Dental worker, including dentist	—	6
Embalmer/morgue technician	1	2
Emergency medical technician/paramedic	—	12
Health aide/attendant	1	15
Housekeeper/maintenance worker	1	12
Laboratory technician, clinical	16	16
Laboratory technician, nonclinical	3	—
Nurse	23	34
Physician, nonsurgical	6	12
Physician, surgical	—	6
Respiratory therapist	1	2
Technician, dialysis	1	3
Technician, surgical	2	2
Technician/therapist, other than those listed above	—	10
Other health care occupations	—	4
Total	**55**	**136**

sure of the mucous membranes of the mouth, nose, and eyes. Gowns or aprons should be worn during procedures that are likely to produce splashes of blood or other body fluids.

Hands and other skin surfaces should be washed immediately and thoroughly if they are contaminated with blood or other body fluids. Moreover, the hands should be washed immediately after gloves are removed. Chemical germicides described as "tuberculocidal" (i.e., able to kill the bacterium that causes tuberculosis) are recommended for decontaminating spills of blood and other body fluid. Visible material should first be removed, then the area should be disinfected. Gloves should be worn throughout the cleaning and disinfecting procedure.

All healthcare workers should take precautions to prevent injuries caused by needles, scalpels, and other sharp instruments or devices during procedures. Precautions should also be used when cleaning used instruments, during disposal of used needles, and when handling sharp instruments after procedures. To prevent needlestick injuries, needles should not be recapped, purposely bent or broken by hand, removed from disposable syringes, or otherwise manipulated by hand. After they are used, disposable syringes and needles, scalpel blades, and other sharp items should be placed in puncture-resistant containers for disposal (i.e., "sharps" containers); the puncture-resistant containers should be located as close as practical to the use area. Large-bore reusable needles should be placed in a puncture-resistant container for transport to the processing area.

Saliva has not been implicated in HIV transmission, but mouthpieces, resuscitation bags, or other ventilation devices should be available for use in areas in which the need for resuscitation is predictable. This availability will minimize the need for emergency mouth to mouth resuscitation. The devices will also reduce transmission of other infectious agents normally transmitted by saliva. Healthcare workers who have lesions expressing fluid or "weeping dermatitis" should refrain from all direct patient care and from handling patient-care equipment until the condition resolves. Such lesions may permit the passage of HIV into the worker's bloodstream.

Pregnant healthcare workers are not known to be at greater risk of contracting HIV infection than nonpregnant healthcare workers; however, if a healthcare worker develops HIV infection during pregnancy, the fetus is at risk of infection through perinatal transmission. Because of this risk, pregnant healthcare workers, like all other healthcare workers, should strictly adhere to the universal precautions.

Implementation of universal blood and body fluid precautions for all patients eliminates the need for use of the isolation category of "Blood and Body Fluid Precautions" previously recommended by the CDC for patients infected with blood borne pathogens. Isolation precautions should be used as necessary if associated conditions, such as infectious diarrhea or tuberculosis, are diagnosed or suspected.

 ## Precautions for Invasive Procedures

An invasive procedure is a surgical entry into tissues, cavities, or organs for repair of major traumatic injuries. It includes treatment in an operating or delivery room, emergency department, or outpatient settings, including both physicians' and dentists' offices; cardiac catheterization and angiographic procedures; a vaginal or cesarean delivery or other invasive obstetric procedure during which bleeding may occur; and the manipulation, cutting, or removal of any oral tissues, including tooth structures, during which bleeding occurs or the potential for bleeding exists. The universal blood and body fluid precautions, combined with the precautions listed here, should be the minimum precautions for all such invasive procedures.

All healthcare workers who participate in invasive procedures must routinely use appropriate barrier precautions to prevent skin and mucous membrane contact with blood and other body fluids of all patients. Gloves and surgical masks must be worn for all invasive procedures. Protective eyewear or face shields should be worn for procedures that commonly result in the generation of droplets, splashing of blood or other body fluids, or the production of bone chips.

Gowns or aprons made of materials that provide an effective barrier should be worn during invasive procedures that are likely to result in the splashing of blood or other body fluids. All healthcare workers who perform or assist in vaginal or cesarean deliveries should wear gloves and gowns when handling the placenta or the infant until blood and amniotic fluid have been removed from the infant's skin, and they should wear gloves during postdelivery care of the umbilical cord.

If a glove is torn or a needlestick or other injury occurs, the glove should be removed and a new glove used as promptly as patient safety permits. The needle or instrument involved in the incident should also be removed from the sterile field. Should an accident occur, the therapies discussed next may be instituted. Table 7.2 presents a brief summary of some of the universal precautions.

 ## Initial Therapy

Healthcare organizations should make available to workers a system that includes written procedures for prompt reporting, evaluation, counseling, treatment, and follow-up of occupational exposures that may place healthcare workers at risk for acquiring HIV infection. Employers are also required to establish exposure-control plans, including postexposure follow-up, and to comply with incident reporting requirements mandated by the Occupational Safety and Health Administration (OSHA).

If an occupational exposure occurs, the circumstances and postexposure management should be part of the worker's confidential medical record. Wounds and skin sites in contact with blood or body fluids should be washed with soap and water, and mucous membranes should be flushed with water. Antiseptics may be applied to the wound, but there is little evidence that the use of antiseptics reduces the risk for HIV transmission. The application of caustic agents such as bleach or the injection of antiseptics or disinfectants into the wound is not recommended by public health physicians.

The source-individual and the exposed healthcare worker should then be evaluated to determine the need for postexposure prophylaxis. The exposure should be evaluated for the potential to transmit HIV based on the type of body substance involved and route and severity of the exposure. Exposures to the fluids enumerated above are situations that pose a risk for bloodborne transmission and require further evaluation. For skin exposures, follow-up is indicated if there is evidence of compromised skin integrity. A human bite must be considered as a possible route of exposure for both the bite recipient and a person inflicting the bite. HIV transmission by this route is extraordinarily rare, however.

 ## Postexposure Prophylaxis

Information about primary HIV infection indicates that sys-

TABLE 7.2 Some Universal Precautions in Brief

1. Wash hands immediately and thoroughly before and after all patient or specimen contacts.

2. Handle the blood of all patients as potentially infectious.

3. Wear gloves for potential contact with blood and body fluids containing visible blood, for touching mucous membranes or non intact skin.
   a. Change gloves after each patient contact.
   b. Do not wash or reuse gloves.
   c. Wash hands after removing gloves and before continuing work.
   d. Wear gloves to cover exudative lesions or weeping dermatitis or refrain from patient contact.

4. Wear a mask with patients who have active tuberculosis.

5. Wear protective gloves, eyewear, and mask if there is a potential for aerosol or being splashed with blood or body fluids.
   Examples: • Respiratory therapist suctioning patient
   • Lab technologist working with blood or body fluids
   • Endoscopy
   • Cardiac catheterization
   • Angiography

6. Wear mask, gown, and eye shields when being splashed with blood or body fluids is anticipated.
   Examples: • Surgery (invasive procedures)
   • Emergency trauma

7. Place used needles/syringes in puncture resistant container. **Do not** bend, break, recap, or manipulate needle in any way.

8. When cleaning up blood spills, wear gloves and use an approved germicide or bleach diluted 1:10. Wipe up the spill with disposable towels.

9. Handle all linen soiled with blood and body fluids as potentially infectious.

10. Locate resuscitation equipment where respiratory arrest is predictable. Eliminate the need for mouth-to-mouth resuscitation.

11. Pregnant healthcare workers are not known to be at greater risk of contracting HIV/HBV infection than those who are not pregnant.

12. Specimens and blood should be clearly labeled so that transport and laboratory personnel are aware of what they are handling and can take special care.

13. Disposable items used in handling specimens should be incinerated or disposed of after procedures for disposal of patients' infectious wastes are followed.

14. Reusable items must be sterilized in the same way as items contaminated with hepatitis B virus.

15. Waste management: Universal Precautions are not intended to change waste management programs previously recommended by the CDC for healthcare settings.

Body Fluids to Which Universal Precautions Apply
- Blood
- Body fluids with or without visible blood
- Semen
- Vaginal secretions
- Cerebrospinal fluid
- Synovial fluid
- Pleural fluid
- Peritoneal fluid
- Pericardial fluid
- Amniotic fluid

temic infection does not occur immediately, but rather leaves a brief "window of opportunity" during which postexposure prophylaxis may be introduced. Animal studies and laboratory research indicates that dendritic cells of the mucosa and skin are the initial targets of HIV infection or have an important role in initiating HIV infection of T cells in regional lymph nodes. Therefore, initiating antiretroviral prophylaxis soon after exposure may prevent or inhibit systemic infection by limiting the proliferation of virus in the target cells.

In most studies, azidothymidine (AZT), also called zidovudine (ZDV), is the antiretroviral agent used for prophylaxis. Other agents such as dideoxycytidine (ddC) and dideoxyinosine (ddI) have been also found effective. Data are not yet available that directly support the addition of other antiretroviral drugs to AZT to enhance the effectiveness of the prophylaxis. However, other drugs can be considered for use, including lamivudine (also called 3TC) and zalcitavine (zal-sit'a-veen). These have been recommended for inclusion in regimens that include AZT. In addition, a protease inhibitor can be used as a third drug for prophylaxis following high-risk exposures, as Chapter 8 explores.

The duration of postexposure prophylaxis is usually four weeks. During this period an important goal is to encourage and facilitate compliance with the drug regimen. Toxicity and the occurrence of side effects are important considerations because they limit compliance with treatment regimens. Unfortunately, all the antiretroviral agents have been associated with side effects, including gastrointestinal upsets such as nausea and diarrhea. In addition, the protease inhibitors may have drug interactions when used with certain other drugs. Therefore, careful evaluation of other medications must be performed. If the HIV status of the source-individual is unknown at the time of exposure, use of prophylaxis should be decided on a case by case basis after considering the type of exposure and the likelihood of HIV infection in the source-individual.

Investigations of healthcare workers suffering occupational exposures to HIV have been performed in France, Italy, and the United States. Results reported in 1995 indicate that AZT could be used to decrease the risk for HIV infection by 81 percent following percutaneous exposure to HIV-infected blood. The study was a retrospective case-control study, meaning that results were assessed from previous incidents rather than from planned experiments. Also, the number of case-patients was small, and the individuals came from separate populations. Some incidents were reported anecdotally.

A more substantial study completed in 1996, showed that postexposure prophylaxis with AZT decreases the risk of HIV infection by an estimated 79 percent in workers exposed to infected blood. Researchers determined that the risk of HIV transmission to a healthcare worker was greatest when the worker suffered a deep injury caused by a device visibly contaminated with a patient's blood. Alternately, transmission occurred when a needle became inserted directly into the worker's vein or artery. Moreover, investigators found elevated risk among workers exposed to the blood of patients having a terminal illness, probably reflecting the large amount of virus found in the blood late in the course of disease.

Two situations may require special consideration. First, the virus from the source-individual may be resistant to antiretroviral drugs. This finding will alter the regimen of drugs used. Second, if the healthcare worker is pregnant, full information should be provided about the potential benefits and risks associated with the use of antiretroviral drugs to the worker and her unborn child. This information will permit her to make an informed decision regarding the use of postexposure prophylaxis. For example, the first trimester is the period of maximal risk for damage to the fetus. The safety and tolerability of the drug or drug combination in pregnancy must also be considered.

At this writing, over 1500 cases of AIDS involving a healthcare worker have been investigated. A relatively small number developed HIV infection in the weeks after their exposure. These observations indicate that for healthcare workers there is a small risk of occupational exposure. The universal precautions explained in this chapter minimize the risk still further.

 ## The Bloodborne Pathogens Standard

The Occupational Safety and Health Administration (OSHA) has issued a Bloodborne Pathogens Standard designed to protect the lives of healthcare workers and ensure that they avoid serious and deadly diseases. Employers who demonstrate their willingness to comply with the standards show concern for their employees and assure that healthcare workers are protected. Employees have the responsibility to remain informed and educated.

The purpose of the Bloodborne Pathogens Standard is to protect healthcare workers from exposure from HIV as well as other bloodborne pathogens such as hepatitis B virus. Under the standard, personal protective equipment must be provided at no cost to the employee. It must be available in the appropriate size and be readily accessible. Gloves must be worn when it is reasonably anticipated that the healthcare worker will have contact with blood, saliva, nonintact skin, or mucous membranes. Hand washing is required after the removal of gloves or other personal protective equipment. A mask, in combination with an eye protection device, should be worn whenever spray, splatter, or droplets of blood or other body fluids may be generated. A fresh mask is indicated for each patient or after one-hour's wear during lengthy procedures, or if it becomes wet during treatment.

Annual retraining is required to keep the awareness level high. A medical record stating the hepatitis B vaccination status of each employee should be maintained by the employer. The hepatitis vaccine must be provided at no cost to the employee.

When an occupational exposure incident occurs, it must be documented in the medical record together with the date of the incident, results of testing after the incident, and the written statement of the healthcare professional that the employee has been informed of the results of testing. These are but a few of the numerous standards that have been set up by OSHA. The full text of regulations can be obtained by contacting OSHA publications office at telephone (202) 219-4667 or through any regional office.

Questions

1. Summarize the methods by which HIV can be transmitted from infected patients to healthcare workers.

2. Describe some of the Universal Precautions used to reduce the likelihood of HIV transmission in the healthcare community.

3. Explain some considerations that reduce or increase the possibility of HIV transmission to healthcare workers from AIDS patients.

Chapter Eight

Diagnosing HIV Infection and AIDS

Review and Preview

Thus far, we have progressed rather deeply into the study of human immunodeficiency virus (HIV) infection and acquired immune deficiency syndrome (AIDS). We studied AIDS in the context of other diseases and explored the structure and replication process of the virus that causes this dread disease. Furthermore, we examined the immune system in depth, because it is responsible for resistance to disease and is the primary focus of infection by HIV. We proceeded to summarize how HIV affects the helper T cells of the immune system, then went on to define some symptoms of patients with HIV infection or AIDS. A rather lengthy discussion outlined some of the opportunistic illnesses that occur in the AIDS patient.

An important factor in dealing with the AIDS epidemic is understanding how the disease spreads in the community, so we devoted an entire chapter to discussing the modes of HIV transmission: sexual means, blood to blood mechanisms, and placental transfer from mother to child. We then talked about how transmission can be prevented. For instance, certain safer sex practices and some practices for injection drug users can interrupt HIV transmission. Among the latter are syringe exchange programs. Drug therapy with AZT during the pregnancy has been valuable in breaking the chain of transmission between mother and child.

In Chapter 7 we highlighted the special dangers for healthcare workers, and precautions they must observe for avoiding HIV transmission through percutaneous injury or by mucocutaneous exposure. Research studies have shown that the average risk of HIV transmission after percutaneous exposure to HIV-contaminated blood is approximately 0.3 percent. After a mucocutaneous exposure, the average risk for HIV transmission is 0.09 percent. Among the factors that affect the risk for HIV transmission are the quantity of blood to which a healthcare worker is exposed, the patient's state of illness, and the worker's own state of health.

A major effort has been made by public health agencies to reduce the likelihood of such transmission. The principles underlying this effort are called Universal Precautions. They include barrier precautions, including the use of gloves, masks, and protective eyewear to prevent exposure during contact with blood and other bodily fluids. Special precautions to prevent injuries by needles, scalpels, and other sharp instruments are included in the Universal Precautions. Recommendations from health agencies also indicate the type of therapy that should be used if a healthcare worker does indeed suffer an exposure.

This chapter describes some of the diagnostic methods available to determine whether a person has acquired HIV after an exposure to contaminated body fluid has taken place. This study begins with some of the health history factors that may influence the final diagnosis. Then we will proceed to laboratory testing and summarize the various indicators pointing to the presence or absence of HIV in the patient's tissues. Since 1985, the antibody tests have been used as criteria for infection because when HIV has entered the body the immune system responds with anti-HIV antibodies. Modern technology has also made available tests to determine whether HIV itself is present in the body. One test for proviral DNA is available, and a second test has been developed that detects the RNA of HIV. Both tests rely on first amplifying the nucleic acid present and using a gene probe to detect the amplified nucleic acid. We will see how both of these work as diagnostic tools.

Introduction

Diagnostic procedures for HIV infection and AIDS are key aspects in the public health response to the AIDS epidemic. These procedures include evaluating the results of clinical findings during a physical examination and analyzing the patient's blood samples for the presence of HIV antibodies and/or signs of the virus itself. Many diagnostic procedures are highly sophisticated applications of modern technologies. They represent an elegant application of the fruits of contemporary research.

 ## Health History and Physical Examination

The diagnostic examination should begin with a review of the patient's health history to establish baseline information about health problems that may have led to HIV infection. A physician should also evalutate the stresses in the patient's life, the status of immunizations for various diseases, as well as practices that may place the patient at high risk for transfer of human immunodeficiency virus (HIV). The physician should refer the patient for counseling or social services if necessary.

The physician will want to know whether the patient has had previous infections such as tuberculosis, because this disease is commonly associated with HIV infection. Any instances of herpesvirus or cytomegalovirus infections, fungal infections, and/or protozoal infections will also be noted, inasmuch as they are common opportunistic illnesses associated with AIDS. The health history should also include information on sexually transmitted diseases such as gonorrhea, syphilis, and chlamydia, because damage of the genital organs as a result of these diseases can encourage the transmission of HIV infection.

Travel, occupational, and residential circumstances should also be noted because they often contribute to the development of opportunistic illnesses. For example, a person living in the southwestern United States and exposed to environmental dust may be in danger of developing coccidioidomycosis (kok"-sid-i-oi'do-my-co-sis). Moreover, patients exposed to polluted water also may be exposed to the protozoa that cause cryptosporidiosis.

The health history will also focus on the immunizations a patient has had because the physician may advise updating and administering vaccines to prevent onset of secondary diseases. The health history should include information on any mental illnesses and/or hospitalizations to determine whether crisis intervention will be necessary should HIV infection progress to AIDS. It is also valuable to discuss any living and social conditions that may influence the development of HIV infection and encourage progression to AIDS. For example, if the patient has a pet cat, exposure to *Toxoplasma* may occur, and toxoplasmosis may ensue.

The health history will also review any recent symptoms experienced by the patient. For instance, night sweats, unexplained fever, unintentional weight loss, recurring fatigue, and unexplained swelling of the lymph nodes may reflect early signs of HIV infection. Other symptoms may be related to the early signs of opportunistic illnesses. For example, difficulty in swallowing and pain in the esophagus may be signs of *Candida albicans* infection, and unexplained diarrhea may be a sign of infection with *Cryptosporidium* (krip"-to-spor-id'i-um). The health history examination will also reveal any neurologic symptoms experienced by the patient, including headache, memory loss, listlessness, and mood swings. Any of these could be a sign of HIV infection.

The diagnosis of AIDS then focuses on physical examination of the patient. A standard measurement of body temperature and inspection of the oral cavity may show that systemic infection is present; sores of the mouth may be related to oral candidiasis, hairy leukoplakia (lu-ko-pla'ke-ah), or Kaposi's sarcoma. Inspection of the lymph nodes will reveal any swelling; and a lung examination will reveal whether any pneumonia is present.

 ## The T Cell Count

The second major approach to AIDS diagnosis is through laboratory testing. This testing reflects the infection of the cells of the immune system and the body's response with HIV antibodies.

A standard laboratory test is performed to count the number of helper T cells (also known as CD4+ cells). Determination of the helper T cell count reflects the progression of the disease. Normally, the count of helper T cells is about 800 to 1000 per cubic millimeter of blood. As this count drops, various stages of HIV infection are reached. For instance, a count of 500 per cubic millimeter indicates that the loss of helper T cells is serious and that antiretroviral therapy should begin. When the count reaches 200 per cubic millimeter, researchers recommend that anti-*Pneumocystis* therapy be instituted to prevent the development of *Pneumocystis* pneumonia. When the count reaches 50 per cubic millimeter, statistics indicate that progression to AIDS is has occurred (if AIDS has not already been diagnosed as a result of opportunistic illness).

 ## The HIV Antibody Test

One of the most important criteria for HIV infection is determining whether a person is producing anti-HIV antibodies. The body's immune system synthesizes these antibodies on entry of the virus to the body. Antibody tests are screening procedures that measure the presence or absence of antibodies but do not give information on the amount of antibody present.

The ELISA Test

The primary screening test for HIV infection is a laboratory test called the enzyme-linked immunosorbent assay (ELISA). The ELISA test is considered a very sensitive test, and it is exceptionally accurate although not 100 percent efficient.

The ELISA test is performed in a semiautomatic fashion using proteins derived from HIV cultivated in the laboratory in human cells. These proteins are known as antigens because they can stimulate an immune response in the body. The antigens are chemically bound to the bottoms of tiny wells on a plastic slide referred to as a microtiter plate. After the patient's blood is obtained, the fluid portion, the serum, is separated from the blood. It is diluted and added in various dilutions to the wells containing HIV antigens. The plate is incubated, and the excessive serum is removed. If anti-HIV antibodies were present in the serum, they reacted with and bound to the HIV antigens during the incubation period. If there were no antibodies in the serum, no antibodies bound to the antigens. Figure 8.1 illustrates this principle.

At this point, another antibody is added to the wells. This is an anti-human antibody—that is, an antibody that will react with human antibodies. The anti-human antibody is linked to an enzyme called peroxidase. The microtiter plate is incubated at a warm temperature. If anti-HIV antibodies are present in the wells (as a result of binding with HIV antigens), the anti-human antibodies will react with them, and the peroxi-

dase enzyme will gather in the wells. If there were no anti-HIV antibodies in the wells (because there were none in the serum), then no reaction with the anti-human antibodies will take place.

Now a chemical substance reacting with the peroxidase enzyme is added to the wells. This substance is called a substrate. If the enzyme is present, it reacts with the substrate, and the substrate changes color. This color change can be detected on a color-sensing instrument. The color change results in a positive test. Conversely, if there was enzyme present, no color reaction would take place and the instrument would fail to detect a color change. The absence of a color change constitutes a negative test. (Note that no enzyme is present in the well: no anti-HIV antibodies were in the well, because none were in the serum.)

A negative ELISA test is considered a conclusion that no antibodies against HIV exist in the patient. It probably means that the patient has not been infected with HIV. However, a person may not have yet produced enough antibodies for detection by the test. Often the immune system takes about six to eight weeks to produce sufficient anti-HIV antibodies to give a positive test. Indeed, some people infected with HIV do not produce detectable antibodies for a period of 1 or 2 years. Therefore, if there is reason to believe that HIV transmission may have occurred, prudence recommends retesting within a period of weeks.

Furthermore, a positive antibody test does not necessarily mean that a person has HIV infection. Under normal circumstances, the ELISA test will be repeated, and if more than one test returns a positive result, then the overall test will be considered positive. In this case, a confirmatory test called the Western blot analysis will be performed.

Sometimes, individuals tested with the ELISA test yield false-positive results—the individual is uninfected, but the test is positive. This situation occurs because a contaminant may have entered the process and reacted with the anti-HIV antibodies. Alternately, there may have been a mechanical error, such as in the color-sensing device. The Western blot assay should rectify this situation.

The Western Blot Assay

The Western blot assay, another antibody test, is more expensive and more difficult to perform than the ELISA test, but its results are more reliable. Although the results are not 100 percent true, they approach 99.9 percent accuracy.

To perform the Western blot assay, HIV antigens are separated from one another through a process called gel electrophoresis (e"-lec-tro-phor-e'sis). In this process, an electric current is placed within the gel on a slide, and the current causes a mixture of the HIV antigens to separate. The large HIV antigens move slowly through the gel, whereas the small antigens move quickly, thus separating the antigens according to size, based on their molecular weight.

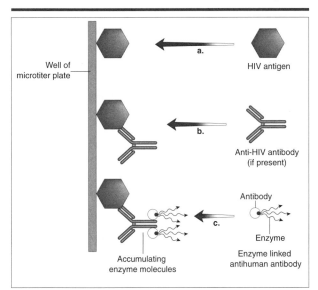

FIGURE 8.1 How the ELISA test works. (a) HIV antigens are bound to the walls of wells in the microtiter plate. (b) Blood serum from the patient is obtained, diluted, and added to the wells. If anti-HIV antibodies are present, they bind to the HIV antigen on the wall. (c) Enzyme-linked antihuman antibodies are added to the well. If anti-HIV antibodies are present on the wall, they link to the enzyme-linked antibodies, and enzyme molecules accumulate. When a reacting substance is added, the enzyme will cause it to change color, indicating a positive test.

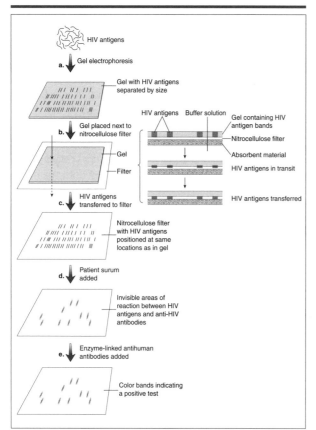

FIGURE 8.2   How the Western blot assay works. (a) HIV antigens from lab-cultivated HIV are separated according to size by the process of gel electrophoresis. (b) The gel is placed next to nitrocellulose paper. (c) The antigens move into the filter, positioning themselves at the same location as in the gel. (d) A sample of the patient's serum is mixed with the paper. If anti-HIV antibodies are present, they will bind with some of the antigens. (e) Enzyme-linked antihuman antibodies are added to the paper. Enzyme molecules accumulate if the anti-HIV antibodies are present. When a reacting substance is added, the enzyme molecules cause a color change, indicating a positive test.

Then the antigens are transferred ("blotted") onto strips of membrane made of a chemical compound called nitrocellulose. Next the patient's serum is mixed with the nitrocellulose membrane containing the HIV antigens, as Figure 8.2 shows. If anti-HIV antibodies are present in the serum, the different antibodies will bind to the various HIV antigens.

Now anti-human antibodies linked to peroxidase enzymes are added to the strip. The antibodies will react with any anti-HIV antibodies bound to the HIV antigens and carry enzyme molecules along with them. Enzyme molecules will thus accumulate (as in the ELISA test). When the reacting substrate is added, it will change color wherever the anti-human antibodies and their linked enzymes have gathered. (And of course, where the anti-HIV antibodies are present.) A set of bands show up in the gel indicating the presence of var-

ious anti-HIV antibodies. Alternately, a radioactive substance can be used with the anti-human antibodies, and the bands will show up on x-ray film as dark smudges, somewhat similar in appearance to a supermarket barcode.

By performing the Western blot assay, the technologist can determine which types of anti-HIV antibody are present in the serum. For example, the test detects antibodies that react with the core proteins of HIV (which are antigens) and with enzyme proteins functioning in viral replication (also antigens). Various health organizations, such as the American Red Cross, require that a positive Western blot assay display antibodies reacting with antigens from at least three major antigen groups.

Because the Western blot assay detects a number of different antibodies in the patient's serum, it is more specific than the ELISA test. However, the Western blot assay is less sensitive than the ELISA test, meaning that it cannot identify all specimens having HIV antibodies. Thus, the ELISA test is a better screening test, and the Western blot assay is a better confirmatory test.

To summarize the above, a three-step process is performed to detect anti-HIV antibodies:

1. An ELISA test is performed on the serum sample. If it is negative, a diagnosis of "negative" is returned and the patient is considered not to have HIV infection. (Remember, however, that infection may have taken place but antibodies may not have yet been produced.)

2. If the ELISA test is positive, it is repeated on the same serum sample. If the second test result is negative, a diagnosis of "negative" is returned.

3. If the person's serum produces two positive ELISA tests, the Western blot assay is performed on the same serum sample. If the test result is negative, the person is designated HIV negative. (In the jargon of the laboratory, the patient has failed to seroconvert.) If the Western blot assay is positive, then a diagnosis of "positive" is returned, and the individual is considered to have HIV infection. (The person has seroconverted.)

If the Western blot test cannot be interpreted due to some laboratory error or other infection present, then an "indeterminate" diagnosis is reported, and the individual is requested to report for another test in a month.

The DNA Viral Load Test

Other HIV antibody tests are available but we shall not consider them here. Rather we shall consider a direct test for HIV. It is called the viral load test because it detects the actual presence and amount of HIV in the blood. The viral load is particularly important early in the infection before the antibodies against HIV have appeared.

The viral load test uses a laboratory procedure called the

TABLE 8.1 Information Gained from RNA Viral Load Testing When Various Clinical Conditions Are Present

Clinical Indication	Information	Use
Syndrome consistent with acute HIV infection	Establishes diagnosis when HIV antibody test is negative or indeterminate	Diagnosis
Initial evaluation of newly diagnosed HIV infection	Baseline viral load "set point"	Decision to start or defer therapy
Every 3–4 months in patients not on therapy	Changes in viral load	Decision to start therapy
4–8 weeks after initiation of antiretroviral therapy	Initial assessment of drug efficacy	Decision to continue or change therapy
3–4 months after start of therapy	Maximal effect of therapy	Decision to continue or change therapy
Every 3–4 months in patients on therapy	Durability of antiretroviral effect	Decision to continue or change therapy
Clinical event or significant decline in CD4+ cells	Association with changing or stable viral load	Decision to continue, initiate, or change therapy

polymerase chain reaction (PCR). The PCR acts as a molecular copy machine. It takes a strand of nucleic acid (such as RNA or DNA) and multiplies it billions of times, thereby amplifying it so that enough is available for detection purposes.

To begin the determination, a number of helper T cells are obtained from the patient's bloodstream. Then the cells are broken open to release their intracellular contents. If the person has been infected with HIV, the virus will have entered the cells and its RNA will have served as a template for the synthesis of DNA. The DNA, known as the provirus, will have integrated to the cell's nucleus. Locating this proviral DNA is the objective of the viral load test using the PCR.

Once the cells have been disrupted, the nuclear material is collected, and the PCR is performed. In a highly sophisticated machine, the double-stranded DNA is unwound to yield single strands of DNA. Then a special heat-resistant enzyme call *Taq* polymerase is added. (The enzyme is obtained from the bacterium *Thermus aquaticus*.) A strand of primer DNA, which recognizes the HIV DNA, is added to begin the elongation, and nucleotides are added to the mixture. Then the mixture is heated. At high temperature, the *Taq* polymerase combines nucleotides to form a strand of DNA complementary to the single strands of DNA, adding them onto the primer DNA one nucleotide at a time. When the mixture is cooled, the new and old strands combine to form new double-stranded DNA molecules. Now the number of DNA molecules has doubled.

Next, the DNA molecules are heated, and they unwind once again. The *Taq* polymerase and primer are added, nucleotides are mixed in, and new strands of DNA are formed, using the bases sequences of the old strands as models. When the mixture cools, the new and old strands combine with one another and the number of DNA molecules doubles yet again. Each new cycle yields another doubling of the DNA molecules. If the proviral DNA was present in the helper T cells, there is now an immense, detectable amount for testing purposes. If proviral DNA was absent (because the person was uninfected), there is no proviral DNA in the mixture of cellular DNA.

Now a gene probe is used. A gene probe is a strand of DNA complementary to the DNA of a provirus, as Figure 8.3 illustrates. The probe will bind to proviral DNA much like a left hand binding to a right hand when the hands are brought together. The gene probe carries a radioactive label. It mingles among the billions of strands of DNA, searching for its complementary DNA, the provirus. If the person is not infected with HIV, this HIV gene probe will not find its proviral DNA match, and the radioactivity will not concentrate anywhere in the available DNA. However, if the person is infected with HIV, the gene probe will locate the proviral DNA and bind to it. This happens billions of times because there are billions of proviral DNA strands after the PCR amplification. Thus, the radioactivity will accumulate in large amounts and send a signal that a match has been made.

The presence of a radioactive signal indicates that proviral DNA is present in the cells and that HIV infection has taken place. Moreover, the intensity of the radioactivity is proportional to the amount of proviral DNA present. Thus, a small amount of radioactivity may indicate that an infection has only recently taken place, while a great deal of radioactivity will indicate much proviral DNA and show that numerous cells have been infected. In this way, the progress of the HIV can be followed.

Early diagnosis of HIV infection is critical not only for detecting whether the disease is present, but also for indicating whether therapy should be instituted. For example, for a pregnant woman and her newborn child, the viral load test indicates whether HIV infection has occurred in the newborn, or whether the antibodies present in the newborn are those derived from the mother.

 The RNA Viral Load Test

New techniques for sensitive detection and accurate quantification of RNA levels in the plasma (blood minus the blood cells) permit the measurement of actual viral particles. These tests are of considerable value in the diagnosis of AIDS. Indeed, RNA testing and viral load determination can be used

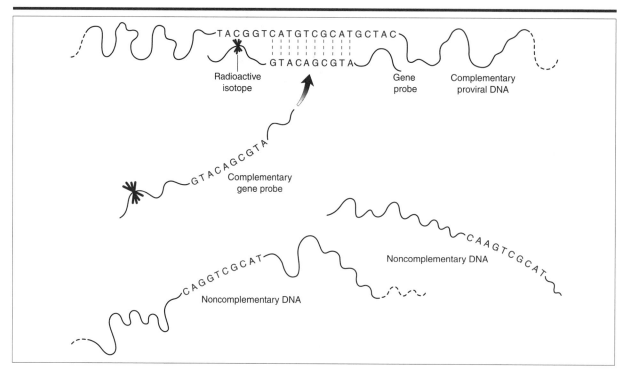

FIGURE 8.3 How a gene probe works. A synthetic fragment of DNA, which is the gene probe, is added to a mixture of DNA molecules. The gene probe reacts only with the DNA molecules that have a complementary code of nitrogenous bases. When a match is found, the radioactive molecules attached to the probe accumulate and send a radioactive signal. If the DNA sought is associated with the provirus of HIV, the test indicates that HIV DNA is present.

to gain information at various points through patients' illnesses, as Table 8.1 indicates. The RNA associated with HIV is found in the blood plasma within circulating virus particles, each particle having two copies of the RNA. The amount of this RNA concentration can be measured (quantitated) to determine the RNA viral load. The test is performed the same way as the DNA viral load test, except that RNA is copied and determined.

Two methods for quantifying the RNA are available. The first is the target amplification method. This method uses the reverse transcriptase RNA polymerase chain reaction to amplify the viral RNA, a variation of the PCR using RNA as the template. The second method is the signal amplification method, which detects the molecular signal sent when a gene probe captures an RNA molecule. The RNA sequences are then quantitated by comparing them to standards.

Versions of both types of assays are now commercially available and approved by the U.S. Food and Drug Administration for assessing the risk of disease progression and for monitoring antiviral therapy in infected individuals. Target amplification assays are more sensitive than signal amplification assays, but only slightly so. Current detection rates are about 400 copies of RNA per milliliter (ml) of blood, but more sensitive versions are constantly being developed.

Quantitative measurements of RNA levels (the viral load) can be expressed in two ways: as the number of copies per ml of RNA associated with HIV, and/or as the logarithm to the base 10 of the number of copies per ml of RNA associated with HIV. Factors influencing the variation seen in RNA assays are based on the performance characteristics of the particular assay. The level of viral infection, as measured by the viral load in the plasma, accurately reflects the extent of viral replication in the patient because viruses produced in the lymphoid tissues are released into the circulation where they can be readily sampled.

During primary infection in adults, when there are numerous target cells and without a substantial host immune response, concentrations of plasma RNA can exceed 10^7 copies per ml. HIV is disseminating widely throughout the body during this period, and many newly infected persons display symptoms of acute viral illness, including fever, fatigue, rash, headache, and pharyngitis. As the antiviral immune responses commence, concentrations of RNA decline rapidly; after a period of fluctuation often lasting six months or more, the plasma RNA levels stabilize at a so-called set point.

Determinants of the set point include the number of susceptible T cells and macrophages available for infection as well as degree of immune activation and the replication rate of the HIV strain infecting the individual. The effects of the host anti-HIV immune response is also a consideration. Once established, set point RNA levels can remain fairly constant for months to years. Studies of populations of individuals suggest a gradual trend toward increasing RNA concentrations as time passes, although the levels can change gradually, abruptly, or hardly at all.

Plasma RNA levels (i.e., the viral load) provide a more powerful predictor of the risk of progression to AIDS and death than does the helper T cell level. For instance, as Figure 8.4 indicates, results from the RNA viral load test can be used to predict the percentage of HIV-infected individuals who will progress to AIDS within 3 years. Indeed, the combined measurement of both T cell levels and viral load provides an even more accurate method to assess the prognosis of HIV-infected individuals.

The level of RNA in the plasma depends on the rate of production and turnover of virus in the circulation. Antiviral therapy disturbs this steady state and begins viral clearance. For example, within two weeks of antiretroviral therapy, the patient's plasma RNA level falls to within 1 percent of its initial values. This decline reflects viral clearance from circulation and increased longevity of T cells. When new rounds of viral replication are blocked by antiretroviral drugs, virus production from infected cells continues for only a short period (about two days).

After the initial rapid decline of plasma RNA, a slower decay of the remaining 1 percent of additional viral RNA is observed. The length of this second phase lasts approximately one to four weeks. Most of the residual virus is thought to arise from infected macrophages lost over a half-life of about two weeks. New rounds of HIV infection are also suppressed, and this suppression appears to be maintained for more than 16 months in most patients adhering to antiretroviral drug therapy.

It must be noted, however, that this interference with HIV replication does not eradicate an established infection. Should the antiretroviral viral therapy be interrupted, rapid rebounds in HIV replication have been observed. In addition, HIV can be isolated from helper T cells obtained from persons undergoing therapy. This is a reservoir of infected T cells that can maintain HIV infection for prolonged periods even when cycles of viral replication are blocked.

 ## Counseling and Testing

As of 1999, 39 of the U.S. states offered anonymous testing, meaning that individuals do not have to give their name to be tested for HIV. All 50 states provide confidential testing, in which one's name is given; and all states have confidentiality laws and regulations to protect this information. For the 5-year period preceding 1999, public health officials noted that the number of anonymous tests declined 26.6 percent and the number of confidential tests increased 2.9 percent. They theorize that anonymous testing has declined because HIV infection is now a more treatable and less stigmatizing disease. Also, new laws and regulations have been enacted to prosecute confidentiality violations.

Testing is valuable because it encourages entry into medical care earlier during the progress of the disease. Infected persons can receive highly active antiretroviral therapy (HAART) using azidothymidine (AZT) and protease inhibitors, which improve the duration of life (Chapter 9). Testing is also useful because after an individual has received a positive result, he or she probably will reduce any risky sexual behaviors that spread HIV. Moreover, HAART may reduce the risk for transmission by lowering the number of infectious viral particles in body fluids of HIV-infected persons. Public health officials estimate that approximately 200,000 persons in the United States are infected with HIV and do not know their HIV status. For these individuals, testing programs can link the individuals to healthcare programs and assist them in adhering to treatment regimens and adopting risk-reduction behaviors.

Before HIV was identified in 1984, researchers were seriously impaired in their efforts to understand AIDS because they could not follow its progress. The development of diagnostic procedures did much to resolve that problem and opened an era of intense research to develop treatments. We will examine the fruits of that research in the next chapter.

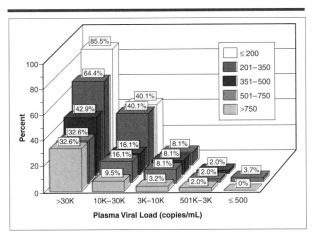

FIGURE 8.4   A comparison of viral load to the percentage of HIV-infected individuals progressing to AIDS within 3 years.

Questions

1. Describe the procedures for the ELISA test and Western blot assay used to detect anti-HIV antibodies in the diagnostic procedure for HIV infection.

2. Summarize the procedure for the DNA viral load test used to detect HIV in the patient.

3. Explain the value of counseling when it is used in conjunction with diagnostic procedures.

Chapter Nine

Treating HIV Infection and AIDS

Review and Preview

When acquired immune deficiency syndrome (AIDS) emerged in American society in 1981, health officials were unsure where the epidemic had come from, where it was centered, and where it might be going. The first observations of the disease had been made a year before, and now the disease appeared to be spreading. As AIDS matured in society, scientists realized that the disease was transmitted by blood and body fluids and that it was affecting broad segments of the national and international populations. Then, in 1984, the human immunodeficiency virus (HIV) was isolated and cultivated by French scientists, and this breakthrough opened a new phase in which AIDS could be characterized as an infectious disease. Scientists studied AIDS in the context of other infectious diseases and began a systematic analysis of HIV, ultimately leading to an understanding of its structure and methods of replication. Other studies led to the realization that HIV had probably emerged from a species of chimpanzee.

As the body of knowledge broadened, scientists came to understand how HIV affects the body and how the symptoms of the HIV and AIDS are related to infection of the helper T cells of the body. Studies were performed on the progression of HIV infection and various theories developed on how HIV destroys the T cells. A case definition for AIDS was developed, and scientists came to appreciate the key roles played by opportunistic illnesses in the deterioration of the patient's health. Research was performed on how AIDS spreads in the community, and we studied various methods in Chapter 5 as we noted the relationship of HIV transmission to sexual transmission, blood to blood transmission, and mother to child transmission.

It is clear that once the transmission methods are understood, measures can be taken to prevent them. Thus, Chapter 6 outlined practices relating to safer sex, safer injection drug use, and safeguards against transmission between mother and child. Because opportunistic pathogens are so important in the progression to AIDS, various methods for avoiding these

organisms were also highlighted.

Chapter 7 considered AIDS in healthcare workers. We noted how transmission occurs in these individuals through exposure to blood and body fluids, but Universal Precautions can be used to interrupt that spread. Through various types of prophylaxis, healthcare workers can further protect themselves. Then, in Chapter 8, we discussed the diagnostic methods available to physicians. The T cell count is an important measure of disease because as the count drops, various stages of HIV infection are reached. The antibody tests such as the ELISA test and the Western blot assay are other indirect criteria for determining whether a person is infected with HIV.

More direct diagnostic tests are used to determine whether HIV is in the body. One test detects the DNA formed by reverse transcriptase after the virus has entered the cytoplasm of the helper T cell. The polymerase chain reaction is used to amplify the DNA so that enough is available for detection, and a gene probe is used to bind to the proviral DNA and denote its presence. A test to detect the RNA of HIV particles in the bloodstream is also available as of this writing. Tests such as these can be used to predict the progression of HIV infection to AIDS and determine whether antiretroviral therapy has been working in the patient.

In this chapter we consider antiretroviral therapy and review some of the available drugs and medications used by physicians. We shall spend considerable time discussing AZT because it has been a standard drug used against HIV since 1987. We shall show how it works and delineate some of its toxic side effects. Because of the latter, alternative therapies such as ddI, ddC, and 3TC are available. Augmenting these therapies are a number of protease inhibitors developed in the 1990s. The combination has been found to reduce significantly the level of HIV infection in the blood. Our discussion will close with some remarks on restoration of the immune system, as this is a primary factor in the patient's return to good health.

Introduction

Viral diseases are more difficult to treat than bacterial or other microbial diseases because viruses lack the complex structures and metabolic patterns that can be interrupted by antibiotics and other medications. Viruses are extraordinarily simple creatures. They have no cell walls or cell membranes, nor do they carry on any metabolic activities. Therefore, few aspects of viral activity can be interrupted by drugs. Furthermore, viruses rely on their host cells for their replication process; therefore, it is difficult to locate drugs that block viral replication without killing the host cell.

Despite these limitations, researchers have developed a number of antiviral drugs that occupy important places in the AIDS regimen of therapy. In addition, there are numerous drugs and medicines that can be used to forestall the opportunistic illnesses that accompany AIDS. We will survey the development and uses of many of those compounds and drugs in this chapter. It is worth noting that new compounds are currently in their testing stage, and many are likely to be available to physicians by the time you read this book.

Because HIV is a retrovirus, AIDS drugs are usually called antiretroviral drugs. To understand the mode of action of antiretroviral drugs, it is important to recall the replication cycle of HIV. This cycle begins when HIV binds with its host cell, the T cell. After the envelope of HIV has united with the membrane of the T cell, the viral nucleocapsid enters the cell's cytoplasm and its protein capsid is broken down by enzymes. Then reverse transcriptase uses the RNA of the virus to produce a DNA molecule. This DNA molecule is called the provirus. The provirus enters the nucleus of the host cell and integrates with its chromosomes.

From this site, the proviral DNA encodes enzymes to compose new RNA molecules and new protein capsids for new viruses. The RNA fragments are enclosed in the capsids, and the newly formed nucleocapsids proceed to the membrane of the cell. Here they "bud" through the membrane to acquire their envelopes. In this way, new HIV particles are formed to continue the infection cycle. Antiretroviral therapies target several aspects of the replication cycle. In addition, many of the principles of antiretroviral therapy accrue from the replication cycle of HIV. Table 9.1 summarizes some of the therapy principles promulgated by the Centers for Disease Control and Prevention (CDC) as of 1998.

Azidothymidine (AZT)

Since its first use in 1987, azidothymidine (AZT) has been a mainstay for treating HIV infection and AIDS. (The drug is

---

TABLE 9.1 Some CDC Principles of Antiretroviral Therapy

1. Ongoing HIV replication leads to immune system damage and progressive AIDS. HIV infection is always harmful, and true long-term survival free of clinically significant immune dysfunction is unusual.

2. Plasma HIV RNA levels indicate the magnitude of HIV replication and its associated rate of CD4+T cell destruction, whereas CD4+T cell counts indicate the extent of HIV-induced immune damage already suffered. Regular, periodic measurement of plasma HIV RNA levels and CD4+T cell counts is necessary to determine the risk for disease progression in an HIV-infected person and to determine when to initiate or modify antiretroviral treatment regimens.

3. As rates of disease progression differ among HIV-infected persons, treatment decisions should be individualized by level of risk indicated by plasma HIV RNA levels and CD4+T cell counts.

4. The use of potent combination antiretroviral therapy to suppress HIV replication to below the levels of detection of sensitive plasma HIV RNA assays limits the potential for selection of antiretroviral drugs to inhibit virus replication and delay disease progression. Therefore, maximum achievable suppression of HIV replication should be the goal of therapy.

5. The most effective means to accomplish durable suppression of HIV replication is the simultaneous initiation of combinations of effective anti-HIV drugs with which the patient has not been previously treated and that are not cross-resistant with antiretroviral agents with which the patient has been treated previously.

6. Each of the antiretroviral drugs used in combination therapy regimens should always be used according to optimum schedules and dosages.

7. The available effective antiretroviral drugs are limited in number and mechanism of action, and cross-resistance between specific drugs has been documented. Therefore, any change in antiretroviral therapy increases future therapeutic constraints.

8. Women should receive optimal antiretroviral therapy regardless of pregnancy status.

9. The same principles of antiretroviral therapy apply to HIV-infected children, adolescents, and adults, although the treatment of HIV-infected children involves unique pharmacologic, virologic, and immunologic considerations.

10. Persons identified during acute primary HIV infection should be treated with combination antiretroviral therapy to suppress virus replication to levels below the limit of detection of sensitive plasma HIV RNA assays.

11. HIV-infected persons, even those whose viral loads are below detectable limits, should be considered infectious. Therefore, they should be counseled to avoid sexual and drug-use behaviors that are associated with either transmission or acquisition of HIV and other infectious pathogens.

also known by its trade names of zidovudine [ZDV] and Retrovir.) AZT is very close in chemical structure to a nucleotide building block of DNA known as thymidine. Thus, when AZT is present in abundance, the cell often selects the AZT molecule in place of the thymidine molecule and uses the AZT molecules to synthesize DNA molecules during the formation of the provirus.

However, the AZT molecule cannot combine with additional nucleotide molecules because it lacks the reactive chemical group where the next nucleotide normally would attach. Therefore, the assembly of a DNA molecule comes to a halt, as shown in Figure 9.1. AZT is therefore known as a "chain terminator," because it brings to an end the construction of the DNA chain of nucleotides. The overall effect is to inactivate any further DNA synthesis and, in effect, prevent the construction of the provirus.

It should be clear that if AZT were incorporated into the host cell DNA, the cellular synthesis of DNA would also come to an end and the cell would die. Unfortunately several types of cells, including bone marrow cells, are susceptible to the deleterious effects of AZT because DNA synthesis is going on at a high rate while red and white blood cells are rapidly being produced. In the presence of AZT, cell multiplication and duplication is interrupted, and the level of red blood cells can fall drastically. For this reason, anemia (a serious lack of red blood cells) is a common side effect of AZT therapy. Among the other side effects of AZT therapy are nausea, vomiting, malaise, and headache. Scientists have isolated HIV strains resistant to AZT from some infected individuals. This resistance is presumably due to mutations that HIV undergoes in its continuing evolution.

It should be noted that AZT is not regarded as a cure for AIDS. Rather, it is a drug that slows the replication of HIV. Of itself, AZT does not restore immune function; it slows the destruction of helper T cells and retards the progression from HIV infection to AIDS. Moreover, as the level of cell destruction decreases, fewer opportunistic illnesses occur in the patient. Overall, AZT significantly increases the average life expectancy of a person with AIDS.

Because AZT can retard the progression to AIDS, public health officials recommend that individuals should be tested quickly if they may have been exposed to HIV. Then they can begin AZT therapy to help interrupt the further development of the disease. Monitoring the helper T cell count is also valuable (Chapter 8).

Another valuable use for AZT is in women who are HIV-positive and pregnant. Therapy can reduce the possibility of HIV transfer to the offspring. AZT therapy has also been used in infected children. These children, who normally acquire HIV from infected mothers, display brain disease. Most children treated with AZT demonstrate improvement, as evidenced by improved appetite, weight gain, and higher T cell counts. In addition, mental function improves, verbal and motor skills increase, and brain involvement appears to slacken.

The cost of AZT is substantial, usually several thousand dollars per year for each person. Treatment regimens demand that a patient take the drug every few hours, but recent studies indicate that lower doses may be just as effective.

AZT is one of a group of drugs called nucleoside analogs. Nucleoside analogs are compounds that resemble the nucleosides and the nucleotides used in the synthesis of RNA and DNA. All nucleoside analogs act in essentially the same way as AZT. But differences may occur in the incidence of side effects.

Other Nucleoside Analogs

Other nucleoside analogs have achieved prominence in AIDS therapy. The first is dideoxyinosine (di"-de-oxy-in'o-seen), abbreviated as ddI. As another reverse transcriptase inhibitor, ddI also prevents the synthesis of DNA. Like AZT, this compound can slow the destruction of helper T cells and interrupt the onset of opportunistic illnesses. The drug is commonly recommended for those who find AZT too toxic or who experience further helper T cell deterioration while taking AZT. One drawback is that the drug is poorly absorbed from the gastrointestinal tract, so it must be suspended in an antacid buffer that has a chalky metallic taste. Chewable tablets are difficult to take as well, especially if a person has oral lesions or dental problems. And because it is susceptible to acidic conditions, ddI must be taken on an empty stomach.

As with AZT, some side effects have been associated with ddI. Reduced white blood cell counts often occur, and many

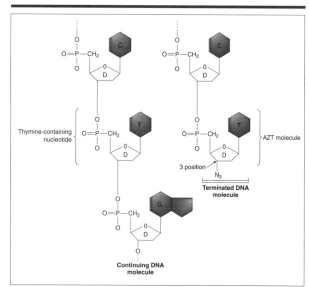

FIGURE 9.1   How azidothymidine (AZT) works. The AZT molecule closely resembles a DNA nucleotide containing thymine. The notable exception is the 3 position, where the AZT molecule contains a triple nitrogen group. After AZT has been incorporated into the DNA molecule, other nucleotides cannot bind to this molecule, and the synthesis of DNA comes to an end.

TABLE 9.2 A Summary of Anti-HIV Drugs

Drug	Mechanism of Action
Azidothymidine (AZT, ZDV, or Zidovudine)	Nucleoside analog; reverse transcriptase inhibitor; nucleotide chain synthesis terminator; increases survival time and reduces incidence of opportunistic infection in AIDS patients; toxic to bone marrow cells; may be used in combination with other drugs in mutiple-drug treatment protcols.
Dideoxycytidine (ddC) Dideoxyinosine (ddI) Stavudine (d4T) Lamivudine (3TC)	Nucleoside analogs; reverse transcriptase inhibitors; mechanism of action and effects are the same as AZT; may have less toxicity than AZT in some patients; may be used in combination with other drugs in multiple-drug treament protocols.
Efavirenz Nevirapine Delavirdine	Nonnucleoside reverse transcriptase inhibitors (NNRTIs); bind directly to the transcriptase and disrupt the catalytic site; do not compete with nucleosides; may be used in combination with other drugs in multiple-drug treatment protocols.
Indinavir Nelfinavir Ritonavir Saquinavir	Protease inhibitors; computer-designed peptide analogs designed to bind to the active site of HIV protease, inhibiting processing of viral polypeptides and virus maturation; may be used in combination with other drugs in multiple-drug treatment protocols.

patients experience rash and diarrhea (probably due to the alkaline conditions of the medications). Peripheral nerve damage can also occur especially in the hands and feet. Effects on the pancreas and liver have been documented, but these side effects are rare. One company markets ddI as Videx, another as didanosine.

The third nucleoside analog approved for use is dideoxycytidine (di"-de-oxy-si'ti-deen) abbreviated as ddC. This compound also inhibits reverse transcriptase activity by acting as a chain terminator for DNA. It is often used in combination with AZT, and it may be substituted if severe AZT side effects are experienced. The major side effect of ddC is peripheral neuropathy (nu-rop'ah-thee), an inflammation of the peripheral nerves. First approved for use in 1992, ddC is chemically similar to ddI. It can cause pancreatitis (pancreas inflammation), but this is not usually severe. The commercial name for ddC is Hivid.

Table 9.2 summarizes many of the antiretroviral agents used in anti-HIV therapy. The three nucleoside analogs we have noted appear to have similar effectiveness. The major differences are their toxicities and the ability of HIV to acquire resistance to the drug. AZT, ddI, and ddC are often used in combination rather than individually. In addition, a strain of HIV acquiring resistance to one drug will usually remain susceptible to the others.

Another important nucleoside analog is 3TC, a drug also called lamivudine (lam-iv'u-deen). It is chemically similar to ddC, and it targets reverse transcriptase. This drug has been used together with AZT and a protease inhibitor in the highly active antiretroviral therapy that we discuss below.

A group of drugs closely allied to the nucleoside analogs are the nonnucleoside analogs. These drugs also react with reverse transcriptase but they do not prevent chain elongation.

Rather the nonnucleoside analogs combine directly with reverse transcriptase and prevent it from operating. Among the important drugs in this group are nevirapine (nev-ir'ah-peen), delavirdine (del-ah-vir'deen), and efavirenz (ef-a-vir'enz). Often one of these drugs is used in combination with a nucleoside analog such as AZT or ddI. The effect is to inhibit reverse transcriptase activity by two methods simultaneously.

 Protease Inhibitors

At the conclusion of the HIV replication cycle, complex proteins are broken down into smaller proteins for the use in constructing the viral capsid. The enzyme used to break down the proteins is called protease. During the 1990s, scientists studied the chemical structure of protease and developed a number of inhibitors that would react with and neutralize this enzyme. When the inhibitor is present, complex proteins cannot be processed, and viral capsids cannot be produced. Thus, HIV replication is interrupted.

Protease inhibitors were developed into a number of drugs that have now become widely used in HIV and AIDS therapy. The drugs are valuable because HIV protease is chemically and structurally different from other protease enzymes found in the human body. Therefore, a drug that blocks the protease associated with HIV will not affect the proteases in other body cells. Side effects would thus be limited.

At this writing, a number of protease inhibitors are in widespread use. Among them are saquinavir (Invirase), indinavir (Crixivan), and ritonavir (Norvir). In therapeutic situations, a protease inhibitor is often combined with AZT and 3TC to be used in a form of medication known as highly active antiretroviral therapy (HAART). In one study, the viral load of patients was measured over a period of time, and in each

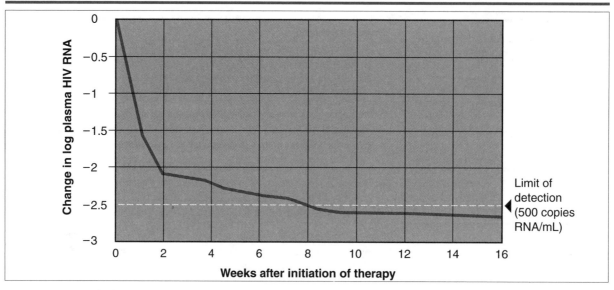

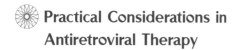

FIGURE 9.2   A graph showing the rate of decline in HIV in the bloodstream following HAART therapy. HIV is measured as copies of HIV RNA, and the rate of decline is expressed as a change in the logarithmic (log) numbers of HIV RNA in the blood plasma.

patient, the level of HIV dropped by 93 percent to 99 percent during the first two weeks of treatment. Moreover, the body eliminated short-lived, infected cells and viral particles. Figure 9.2 uses statistics compiled through 1998 to illustrate the decline of HIV in the bloodstream after using HAART.

Practical Considerations in Antiretroviral Therapy

The most effective methods for preventing HIV infection are those that protect against HIV exposure. Such behaviors as sexual abstinence, consistent and correct use of latex condoms, abstinence from injection drug use, and use of sterile equipment by injection drug users do much to prevent the transmission of HIV. Some healthcare providers have proposed offering immediate antiretroviral therapy to persons who may have been inadvertently exposed to HIV through sexual activity or injection drug use. No data exist on the effectiveness of this therapy. Nevertheless, information about additional physiologic events occurring after HIV exposure suggests that it can take several days for infection to become established in the lymphoid and other tissues. Intervention to interrupt viral replication could prevent an exposure from becoming an established infection.

The frequency, severity, and reversibility of side effects must be weighed against the usefulness of antiretroviral agents for the patient. Adverse events have been recorded from persons with advanced HIV disease, but persons with less advanced disease or uninfected individuals might have different experiences. Although the side effects can be managed, the probability of transmission must be weighed against the risk of severe side effects. In studies with AZT among healthcare workers who have had possible HIV exposure, as many as 35 percent did not complete the full course of therapy, most because of the side effects.

Furthermore, the availability of antiretroviral agents could undermine public health efforts aimed at increasing efforts to change behaviors that prevent HIV exposure because if people perceive that prophylaxis prevents HIV infection, they might increase the frequency of risk behaviors or shift from low risk to high risk activities. Indeed, a 28-day course of antiretroviral agent for a single possible exposure to HIV costs an estimated $600 to $1000, depending on the agent or agents used. This cost is probably more per client than the cost of enrollment in behavioral HIV-prevention programs designed to reduce the likeliness of exposures.

As of the current writing, health officials recommend that postexposure therapy should not be administered routinely or solely at the request of a patient. Patients should not see HAART therapy as a "morning-after pill." Persons with nonoccupational exposures should receive medical evaluations that include HIV-antibody tests at baseline and periodically for at least six months after exposure, usually at intervals of 4 to 6 weeks, 12 weeks, and 6 months. They should be counseled to initiate or resume protective behaviors to prevent additional exposure.

Other Therapies

In the effort to destroy HIV and treat AIDS, numerous other therapies have been developed, and still others are in the process of being developed. One example is soluble CD4. This is a protein identical to the CD4 receptor site at the surface of helper T cells. Produced by genetic engineering methods, soluble CD4 is designed to combine with the envelope of HIV at the spot where the virus normally interacts with the CD4 receptor site of the host cell. Researchers believe that if enough soluble CD4 is present in the bloodstream, the molecules will act as a decoy and attach to the HIV envelope. Thus neutralized, the HIV could not attach to host cells and theoretically, any further infection should be eliminated. Clinical trials with soluble CD4 are currently underway.

Another possible agent for chemotherapy is dextran sulfate, which apparently interferes with viral entry to host cells, though the mechanism is not yet understood. In other countries, dextran sulfate is used as a blood anticoagulant, and its side effects appear to be minimal. However, this drug's effect on HIV is not substantial, so interest in this compound is not acute.

A Chinese herbal is the source of compound Q, also known as GLQ223. Technically the compound is known as tricosanthin. It has shown some preferential activity against HIV-infected macrophages and it appears to block viral replication in host cells. However, serious side effects, including coma, may limit its use.

The envelopes of HIV contain a number of glycoproteins. Disruption of these glycoproteins in the viral envelope is the objective of a drug called castanospermine (cas"-ta-no-sperm 'een). Presumably, this disruption will make the virus unable to infect host cells. Work is continuing on this approach to therapy.

Still another approach to HIV therapy involves antisense molecules. Antisense molecules are synthetic RNA molecules that unite with naturally occurring mRNA molecules produced during the process of protein synthesis. During HIV replication, the provirus integrates to the cell nucleus and encodes mRNA molecules for the production of enzymes and other proteins for viral synthesis. Antisense molecules are specifically designed mRNA molecules that unite with naturally produced mRNA molecules and interfere with their action. The molecules enter the infected cell, and like left hands uniting with right hands, they combine specifically with complementary mRNA molecules. Thus, the mRNA molecules are inactivated, and the synthesis of HIV comes to an end. Therapies using antisense molecules are currently in the developmental stage.

Gene therapy may one day be used to help alleviate the viral load in HIV-infected patients. Trials are now ongoing with genes attached to the DNA of mouse viruses harmless to humans. These mouse viruses have been genetically engineered with HIV genes that encode HIV proteins. The mouse viruses are injected to infected individuals, where they should cause no harm. Researchers believe, however, that the HIV genes will stimulate normal body cells to produce HIV proteins. The proteins would then stimulate the body's immune system to produce anti-HIV antibodies. Presumably, these antibodies will react with HIV in the body and forestall the destruction of helper T cells.

Another form of gene therapy involves HIV particles whose genes for replication have been removed. These mutant HIV particles are combined in test tubes with host T cells from HIV-infected individuals. The mutated viruses enter the cells, then the cells are cultivated and injected back into the patient. The helper T cells contain virus, but the virus cannot reproduce because it lacks the critical genes. However, the infected cells can now stimulate the body to produce a class of immune system cells known as killer T lymphocytes. Hopefully, these cells will react with other HIV-infected cells in the body and destroy those cells.

HIV Mutation and Drug Therapy

As noted previously, the replication of HIV uses an enzyme called reverse transcriptase, which is encoded by the HIV genome. The enzyme is an RNA-dependent DNA polymerase. It synthesizes the single-stranded genome of HIV into a double-stranded DNA molecule during an essential step in the replication cycle of the virus.

However, this DNA polymerase (reverse transcriptase) is unlike that found in the human cell: the DNA polymerase of host cells possesses a 3-prime exonuclease activity that performs a "proofreading" function and repairs errors made during transcription. The reverse transcriptase of HIV lacks this activity. As a result, during the transcription of the HIV genome, numerous transcriptional "errors" occur. These errors give rise to numerous mutations in new viral genomes produced within infected host cells. Estimates of the mutation rate of reverse transcriptase predict that, on average, one mutation is introduced in every one to three HIV genomes produced. More variation is introduced into the replication cycle of HIV because two RNA molecules are present in each virus, and template-switching occurs as the enzyme uses first one RNA molecule then the other to make the DNA.

Many mutations introduced into the HIV genome during the process of reverse transcription will compromise or eliminate the infectivity of the virus. But other mutations are compatible with virus infectivity. In HIV-infected individuals, the frequency with which genetic variants of HIV arise depends in part on the nature of selective pressures acting on the existing variants. Such selective pressures include the anti-HIV immune response, the number of host cells available for viral infection, and the use of antiretroviral drug therapy.

The numerous rounds of HIV replication occurring daily

TABLE 9.3 Some Benefits and Risks of Using Antiretroviral Therapy in HIV-Infected Individuals Before Symptoms Have Developed

Potential Benefits

Control of viral replication and mutation; reduction of viral burden

Prevention of progressive immunodeficiency; potential maintenance or reconstitution of a normal immune system

Delayed progression to AIDS and prolongation of life

Decreased risk of selection of resistant virus

Decreased risk of drug toxicity

Potential Risks

Reduction in quality of life from adverse drug effects and inconvenience of current maximally suppressive regimens

Ealier development of drug resistance

Limitation in future choices of antiretroviral agents due to development of resistance

Unknown long-term toxicity of antiretroviral drugs

Unknown duration of effectiveness of current antiretroviral therapies

in infected individuals generates large numbers of variant viruses, including many that display diminished sensitivity to antiretroviral drugs. A mutation is probably introduced into every position of the HIV genome many times each day within an infected person, and the variants may accumulate within the virus population with successive cycles of virus replication.

This great genetic diversity is probably present before antiretroviral therapy has begun. Indeed, researchers have identified mutants with drug-resistance in HIV-individuals who have never been treated with antiretroviral drugs. Once drug therapy begins, the population of drug-resistant viruses can rapidly predominate. When drugs such as 3TC are used, for example, a single nucleotide change in the HIV gene for reverse transcriptase can confer reductions in drug susceptibility of 100 to 1,000 fold. The antiretroviral activity of drugs used alone is largely abolished within four weeks of initiation of therapy due to the rapid development of drug-resistant variants. For this reason, "cocktails" of drugs (i.e., drug combinations) are advised.

Public health officials caution that the development of drug-resistant mutants is but one drawback to the use of antiretroviral therapy in a patient who has not yet developed symptoms of HIV infection. Other risks, as well as some benefits, are summarized in Table 9.3.

 Therapy in Pediatric HIV Infection

Although the pathogenesis of HIV infection and the principles underlying the use of antiretroviral therapy are similar for all HIV-infected persons, unique considerations exist for HIV-infected infants, children, and adolescents. Most HIV infections in children are acquired perinatally, and most perinatal transmission occurs during or near the time of birth. This timing raises the possibility of initiating treatment in an infected infant during the period of initial HIV infection, as

long as diagnostic tests have defined the infants' infection status early in life. Also, it should be noted that perinatal HIV infection occurs during the development of the infant's immune system (rather than in the mature system in adults). Therefore, both the clinical manifestations of HIV infection and the course of immunologic and virologic markers of infection differ from those for adults.

Treatment of infected children takes into account a prior exposure to AZT, as antiretroviral drugs were used during pregnancy and during the neonatal period for treatment of the mother and/or for preventing perinatal transmission. In addition, the pharmaceutical activities of the drug change during the transition from the newborn period to adulthood, and this change requires specific evaluation of drugs dosages and toxicity in infants and children. Finally, adherence to therapy in

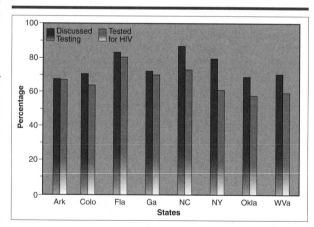

FIGURE 9.3 Results of a CDC survey conducted in eight states showing that when pregnant women discussed HIV and AIDS with their healthcare providers, the great majority agreed to HIV testing. In many cases this testing successfully identified HIV at an early stage in the disease and permitted AZT therapy, which interrupted transmission to their offspring.

children and adolescents requires certain considerations not necessarily applying to adults.

Early identification of HIV-infected pregnant women is crucial for their health and for the care of HIV-exposed and HIV-infected children. This identification is often dependent on counseling with healthcare providers, as Figure 9.3 demonstrates. Knowledge of the mother's HIV status enables HIV-infected women to receive anti-HIV therapy and medical prophylaxis against opportunistic illnesses for their own health. It also encourages use of prophylaxis with AZT during pregnancy and labor, and then with the newborn. Moreover, counselors can chat with infected women about the risks for HIV transmission through breast milk and advise them about potential safe alternatives. Counseling permits prophylaxis against *Pneumocystis carinii* pneumonia to begin in HIV-exposed infants beginning at the age of four to six weeks, according to guidelines set up by the Public Health Service.

Viral diagnostic assays can identify HIV infection in most infants by the age of one month, and in virtually all infected infants by the age of six months. Detection of HIV by culture or by DNA or RNA polymerase chain reaction indicates a possible HIV infection, which should be confirmed by a repeat virologic test on a second specimen as soon as possible. HIV culture is more complex and expensive to perform than nucleic acid analyses, and definitive results may not be available for two to four weeks.

As noted, the viral load in the child's peripheral blood can be determined by using the quantitative RNA assay. A high viral RNA copy number usually persists in the infected children for prolonged periods. Levels are generally low at birth, but they increase to high values by the age of two months, then decrease slowly. This pattern probably reflects the low efficiency of an immature but developing immune system in containing the viral replication. It may also reflect a greater number of HIV-susceptible cells.

Antiretroviral therapy has provided substantial clinical benefits to HIV-infected children who have clinical or immun-ologic symptoms of HIV infection. Studies have demonstrated substantial improvement in neurodevelopment, growth, and immunologic or virologic status after AZT treatment has begun. Similar results have been found with ddI, and 3TC. Clinical trials of symptomatic children who were not previously treated with antiretroviral drugs have demonstrated that combination therapy with either AZT and 3TC or with AZT and ddI is superior to therapy with a single drug. Furthermore, combination therapy that includes a protease inhibitor is superior to therapy with only two nucleoside analogs.

At the current time, combination therapy is recommended for all infants, children, and adolescents. As compared with monotherapy, combination therapy slows disease progression and improves survival; it results in a greater and more sustained virologic response, and it delays the development of viral mutations that allow viruses to resist the drugs used in therapy. Indeed, monotherapy with antiretroviral drugs is no longer recommended, except for AZT monotherapy, which is appropriate when used in infants of indeterminate HIV status during the first six weeks of life. If the infant is identified as being HIV-infected, then the monotherapy should be changed to combination therapy. Aggressive antiretroviral therapy with three drugs is recommended because it provides the best opportunity to preserve immune function and delay the progression of the disease.

 Treatment of Opportunistic Illnesses

Opportunistic illnesses are a key manifestation of AIDS, and treating them is an important objective of the overall regimen of therapy. For *Pneumocystis carinii* pneumonia (PCP), the treatment includes aerosolized pentamidine isethionate (pentam'i-deen i-se-thi'o-nate). Alternatives are trimethoprim (tri-meth'o-prim) combined with sulfamethoxazole (sul-fah-meth-ox'ah-zole), a combination known commercially as Bactrim. Since the beginning of the AIDS epidemic, PCP has

TABLE 9.4 Some Adverse Side Effects Associated with Therapy for Opportunistic Illnesses

Side Effect	Drug Therapy
Bone marrow suppression	Cidofovir, dapsone, ganciclovir, pyrimethamine, rifabutin, sulfadiazine, trimethoprim–sulfamethoxazole, trimetrexate
Diarrhea	Atovaquone, clindamycin
Hepatotoxicity	Clarithromycin, fluconazole, isoniazid, itraconazole, ketoconazole, pyrazinamide, rifabutin, rifampin
Nephrotoxicity	Amphotericin B, cidofovir, foscarnet, pentamidine
Ocular effects	Cidofovir, ethambutol, rifabutin
Pancreatitis	Pentamidine, trimethoprim–sulfamethoxazole
Peripheral neuropathy	Isoniazid
Skin rash	Atovaquone, dapsone, sulfadiazine, trimethoprim–sulfamethoxazole

been the most common AIDS-defining-opportunistic illness, and since 1995, triple combination therapy for HIV infection (i.e., HAART) probably has had a substantial impact on the incidence of PCP and other opportunistic illnesses by slowing the progression of HIV disease. However PCP still occurs among persons who were tested late for HIV or who failed to obtain adequate care. In addition, the incidence of encephalitis due to toxoplasmosis has also decreased. This may have occurred because the medication for PCP also treats toxoplasmosis. Unfortunately, many of the drug medications used against opportunistic illnesses themselves have side effects, as Table 9.4 summarizes.

Two other opportunistic illnesses, herpes simplex and cytomegalovirus (CMV) disease, can also be treated using antiviral therapies. For herpes simplex, the drug of choice is acyclovir, and for CMV disease, it is ganciclovir. Both drugs interfere with the synthesis of DNA in the genome of the virus. For tuberculosis and other mycobacterial diseases, isoniazid and rifampin are effective therapies, as are clarithromycin and azithromycin. Antifungal agents such as amphotericin B are used against such opportunistic illnesses as cryptococcosis, while nystatin and miconazole are useful against *Candida albicans* infections.

Unfortunately, some opportunistic illness are extremely difficult to treat. Cryptosporidiosis, the serious intestinal diarrhea, is one such example of an illness where only marginally effective treatments are available. Otherwise, a wide variety of drugs are available for dealing with opportunistic illnesses. This should encourage HIV-infected patients to seek help and place themselves under the care of a physician. Such treatment has been shown to delay successive bouts of opportunistic illness and lessen the possibility of serious damage to the tissues. Physicians also can help patients feel that they are taking positive steps to fight off AIDS, and this positive mental attitude will help considerably in the long run.

Restoration of the Immune System

The hallmark of HIV disease is the death of massive numbers of helper T cells. The low T cell count almost invariably signals trouble for the HIV patient. Most of the significant damage to the immune system occurs within the first three to six months after infection. During this period, patients usually do not realize that they are infected nor do they have symptoms.

During the early weeks, the immune system is so damaged that the helper T cell population is virtually eliminated. Also, a pool of about 1 million infected cells emerges. This pool stays about the same for about the first year of infection. The available drugs cannot eliminate the infected cells in that pool. Moreover, there is a dramatic depletion of helper T cells of the naive type. Naive cells are young cells that have not yet participated in an immune response. There is also a sharp rise in antibodies against HIV, followed by a drop and then a low

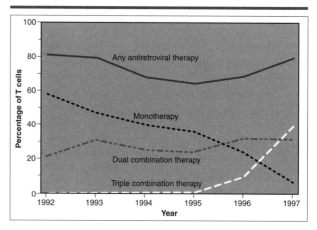

FIGURE 9.4 The number of CD4+ T cells in patients treated with various forms of anti-HIV therapy over a 5-year period. Monotherapy, such as with AZT, can prolong life, but the T cells count drops nevertheless. Dual (two drug) therapy results in a stabilizing T cell count. By comparison, triple combination therapy such as HAART, results in a sharp rise in the T cell count, as shown by statistics gathered over a multiyear period.

level of antibody production. The antibody response is therefore ineffective.

In an uninfected adult, one-third of all T cells are naive (CD4+) helper T cells, another third are memory T cells, and the rest are (CD8+) suppresser T cells. Now HIV enters the picture. Only 2 percent of the surviving T cells are naive CD4+ helper T cells, and 7 percent are memory CD4+ T cells. The remaining 91 percent of all T cells are CD8+ cells. The memory cells are older cells that have encountered antigens and "remember" the same type of microbe if it returns. In the absence of helper T cells or other immune response, HIV particles reside inside the cells of the lymph nodes, tonsils, and spleen. Here they replicate themselves and infect passing CD4+ cells.

Patients taking highly active antiretroviral therapy show signs of immune system improvement, as the graph in Figure 9.4 demonstrates. Their counts of CD4⁺ cell rise and the CD8⁺ population drops back proportionally. These patients do not develop as many illnesses as their immune system fights off the opportunistic microorganisms that cause opportunistic illnesses. In some cases there is a rise in naive CD4⁺ cells, which indicates that patients are making new T cells. In some cases, researchers have reported that their patients are recovering from Kaposi's sarcoma and losing the purple skin blotches that occur in HIV-positive men. This is evidence for a strengthened immune response. Other researchers have shown that the size of the thymus has enlarged in individuals taking HAART. This data is taken as evidence that thymus cells are forming new naive CD4⁺ cells.

The use of antiretroviral therapy, unfortunately, does not

necessarily mean that the immune response will always return to normal. The damage inflicted upon the immune system and its structural elements, the lymphoid tissues, may be permanent. The development of immunocompetent T cells from immature naive cells has not been conclusively demonstrated; it is possible that once lost, the cell responses may not be regained, even if new rounds of HIV infection can be stopped by effective antiretroviral therapy. Similarly, it is not known if the damaged architecture of the lymphoid organs observed in persons with moderate to advanced HIV disease can be repaired following antiretroviral drug therapy.

With this possibility in mind, initiation of antiretroviral therapy before there is extensive immune system damage will be more effective in preserving and improving the ability of HIV-infected persons to mount protective immune responses. It is possible that some improvement in immune function will be observed even in patients who have advanced HIV disease, as opportunistic illnesses appear to occur at less aggressive levels in persons treated with antiretroviral therapy.

The extent to which antiretroviral therapy can restore function represents an essential question for further research. Scientists have found that the development of the immune system is an extremely complex process requiring numerous cell factors, enzymes, and unidentified materials. Reconstituting the immune system may be possible by the transfer of T cells or by the introduction of bone marrow cells. Compounds that enhance the function of normal cells are also being researched, and enhancement factors such as interleukin-2 have attracted interest. To be sure, any treatment that can raise the T cell count to a level of 500 per milliliter of blood is desirable. Full reconstitution of the immune system requires raising the level to between 800 and 1000 T cells per milliliter of blood. Accomplishing this remains a prime objective of contemporary researchers.

Questions

1. Summarize the mode of action and uses of AZT therapy for treating HIV infection and AIDS.

2. Discuss the mode of action of the protease inhibitors and indicate their use in AIDS therapy.

3. Explain some other therapies used against HIV and some therapies used against opportunistic pathogens.

Chapter Ten

AIDS and Society

Review and Preview

And so we come to the end of our pathway of discovery. We have seen how acquired immune deficiency syndrome (AIDS) arrived on the American scene in the early 1980s, and how scientists grappled with the uncertainties relative to its cause. Eventually, however, they isolated the human immunodeficiency virus (HIV) and identified how it is spread among humans. With this information in hand, they could plot strategies to interrupt its transmission and provide the world's population with measures to prevent exposure to the virus. This was particularly important for healthcare workers, who help AIDS patients on a daily basis.

Diagnostic methods are of paramount importance in quelling the spread of HIV because they help identify those who have the disease. We saw in Chapter 8 that antibody determinations and direct viral measurements can be used to discern whether a person is infected with HIV and learn the extent of the infection. The antibody tests are relatively inexpensive and easy to perform, but they can be unreliable if the body has not produced sufficient detectible levels of antibodies. The direct viral load tests give a more accurate view of the extent of infection but are more difficult and much more expensive to perform. Counseling is another essential aspect of the diagnostic procedure.

Another major factor in dealing with the AIDS epidemic is developing suitable treatments. In Chapter 9 we outlined some of the various methods now used in antiretroviral therapy. AZT has been the mainstay in the drug regimen since 1987. This compound interrupts the assembly of the DNA molecule synthesized by reverse transcriptase using the RNA of HIV as a model. However, body cells that synthesize much

DNA are affected severely by AZT. When it is used with other drugs such as 3TC and protease inhibitors, AZT is effective in halting the spread of HIV and in reducing the possibility of a pregnant mother spreading HIV to her offspring. It is important to note that therapies are available to treat the opportunistic illnesses that signal the progression to AIDS. For example, drug therapies are available to halt toxoplasmosis, *Pneumocystis carinii* pneumonia, cryptosporidiosis, cytomegalovirus disease, and other opportunistic illnesses. Unfortunately, antiretroviral therapies are very expensive, which limits their use in nonaffluent communities. Moreover, these therapies may not work well when HIV mutates to a drug-resistant form.

It is abundantly clear that the AIDS epidemic will continue to confront our society in the future. Thus, while considering the science of AIDS, we must also consider the societal issues associated with the disease. The remainder of this book is a brief review of how AIDS affects various groups. We will also focus on the effects of medical care as it impacts the AIDS epidemic and talk about budgeting resources to fight the epidemic. One of the hopes for the future is that scientists will develop an effective vaccine against HIV and AIDS, so we will look at their progress to date. Before the vaccine becomes a reality, however, social science has much to offer in helping individuals change their behavior. Hence, we will identify some places where the social sciences will be valuable in the future. And finally, we will attempt to tie together many of the concepts covered in these chapters and look into the future to predict some of the challenges lying ahead.

Introduction

When AIDS was a mysterious and unexplained illness, it could be understood as a random act of chance or something separate from society. Today, however, scientists understand the mechanics of AIDS, and they realize that its spread is subject to human decisions and social policies. Indeed, many individuals believe that the AIDS epidemic could be halted entirely by social means if they were coercive and extreme.

Although the AIDS epidemic has resulted in terrifying losses of life, and although high numbers of deaths are projected for the future, major medical breakthroughs could bring the AIDS epidemic to a conclusion. Few seriously believe that AIDS will bring an end to Western civilization, even though some did believe this at the beginning of the epidemic. However, AIDS will continue to cause population loss, resource depletion, and psychological and social reactions. It will continue to change the characteristic of human social life.

AIDS will continue to result in high casualty rates among the population until its spread is halted and reversed. Countries of Africa, in particular, will suffer a seriously heavy burden because the prevalence of AIDS is high on that continent. However, the extremely high birth rate in Africa and other epidemic diseases are important factors that will also influence the population numbers.

Economic disruption and resource depletion will continue in many countries, and painful choices in resource allocation lie ahead. Resource depletions may make a society vulnerable to other types of attack. For example, healthcare costs already cause hardship in the United States, where the care of a single AIDS patient often exceeds $100,000 over the course of the disease. This occurs in spite of the estimated $1.5 billion spent annually by the U.S. government on research and education relating to the disease. In addition, the profitability of health insurance organizations will be threatened. The need for personnel and hospital facilities will continue to rise, and the budgeting allotments may force hard choices of new taxes or reductions in other expenditures.

In the psychological and social realm, the AIDS epidemic has the potential for creating political instability in developing nations where public order is already precarious. Like the Black Death in Europe in the 1300s, AIDS could trigger religious movements based in ignorance, as well as scapegoating and paranoia. In emerging nations, the AIDS epidemic could make newly developed democratic institutions vulnerable.

In these societal issues we see some of the debilitating effects of the AIDS epidemic. We will explore other issues as we continue to examine the impact of the AIDS epidemic in the national and the global society.

The AIDS Patient

AIDS is another infectious disease—no more, no less. It is not symbolic of anything. There are no "victims," because there is

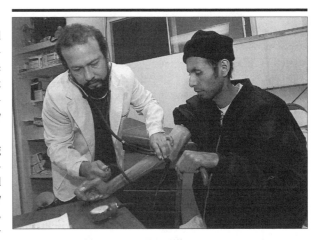

FIGURE 10.1   The AIDS patient carries of a heavy burden of physical, psychological, and social burdens.

no crime. There are no "innocent," because there are no "guilty." And there is no blame, because there has been no intention to cause harm. There are only sick men, sick women, and sick children, all of whom need our help and society's help (Figure 10.1).

To learn that one carries the AIDS virus is to anticipate an inevitable loss of control: the fear of losing friends, neighbors, and perhaps a job, as well as the prospect of losing one's health and quite possibly one's life. In attempting to rebuild his or her world after hearing the electrifying diagnosis of HIV infection, the patient unfortunately tends to swallow whole the popular view of this disease—one's fate is sealed. When the opportunity for creative intervention is defeated, the patient's world becomes wrapped in profound secrecy and anger sets in. The stress of confronting not only one's mortality but also a society that often treats the AIDS patient like a criminal provokes a harsh response.

Many social psychologists believe that the average person has a profoundly negative bias toward AIDS. Normally, the disease not only stigmatizes the patient, but in an odd reversal, the disease itself is stigmatized by its patients, the majority of whom are injection drug users and men who have sex with men. Although people do realize that they will not contract HIV easily, the disease brings to mind things they would prefer not to think about: death, drugs, and anal sex.

AIDS in Women

One of the fastest-growing groups suffering from AIDS is women. Most women are infected through heterosexual contact, and they are often casualties of a political stalemate over how, when, or whether the spouses and lovers of HIV-infected individuals should be told of their exposure to the virus. Many states rely heavily on the expectation that the people who test positive for the virus will inform their sexual partners. However the strategy has failed in many respects, and women at risk for heterosexually transmitted HIV are not informed.

Counselors report that they repeatedly see women who have comforted their husbands or boyfriends through long hospital stays but never learned their partners had AIDS or an illness related to AIDS. They were not told by the attending doctors and nurses that they were at risk themselves. Often these women learn from the grapevine that their partner has died of AIDS. Very often when the women ask why they were not told, the physician answers "we thought you knew."

Among the psychological factors that prevent HIV-infected individuals from revealing their status to their partners are denial, fear of rejection, fear of retaliation, and the loss of confidentiality implicit in directly telling partners of their status. Doctors often have the permission, but not the obligation to notify a partner at risk without divulging the patient's name. There is a growing recognition that many of the women most at risk have been left in the dark, both by AIDS education campaigns and by the haphazard approach to partner notification that exists in many states. Adding to the problem is the reluctance of some gynecologists to accept women with AIDS as patients for regular checkups and routine treatment.

AIDS in Adolescents and Teens

Each year, thousands of new cases of AIDS are reported in young people aged 13 through 21 years. With this in mind, society must realize that AIDS in teens is not limited to under-privileged, inner-city populations. For example, a teenage girl from a small rural community reported that she had had one sexual partner, a young man with hemophilia, whom she knew very well. He did not realize that he had acquired HIV infection from infected blood during a transfusion. And she did not know that he could transmit HIV to her—and thus she became infected at age 16.

Among participants in an adolescent AIDS program, there is usually a wide variation in the number of sexual partners adolescents have. Young women who are infected may have had only one sexual partner. Among boys, same-sex experiences were the leading risk factor for spreading HIV, whether or not the boys considered themselves gay. In addition, HIV transmission is linked to using crack cocaine and engaging in "survival sex" in exchange for money, food, shelter, or drugs.

Many adolescents continue to have sex even after they know they are HIV-positive because they cannot figure out a way to tell their sexual partners, schoolmates, or their family. They are afraid that telling people might cost them their homes or their friends. Counselors advise that the healthy message for physicians is to encourage their adolescent and teenage patients to delay the age of first intercourse and to use condoms whenever they have sex. It is also worth noting that in other industrialized nations, the age at first intercourse is roughly the same as in the United States, but the rates of sexually transmitted diseases are much lower and there is little HIV infection among adolescents. In some of these nations the government provides rigorous health services to teenagers. For example, every teenager in Finland receives a brochure from the government on his or her 16th birthday that portrays adolescent sexuality positively and talks about responsibility while having sexual relations. It also provides a latex condom.

 ## AIDS in the Workplace

Because AIDS is a leading cause of death for Americans between the ages of 25 and 44, the disease impacts heavily on the nation's workforce. Thus, because of their commitment to the community, businesses should be valuable allies in the campaign to educate the public about HIV infection and AIDS.

How well businesses are responding to this challenge was determined in a survey conducted by the U.S. Centers for Disease Control and Prevention (CDC) during 1998. Over 2200 businesses were surveyed from across the country to determine their response to the AIDS epidemic. Forty-three percent of businesses having more than 50 employees reported having a policy in place for an employee with a disability or life-threatening illness such as AIDS. The survey also found that corporate philanthropy was the most common way for businesses to be involved with the AIDS epidemic. Nearly all businesses offered group health insurance, although 5 percent limited or excluded HIV from at least one of the policies offered to employees. The survey further found that 60 percent of business firms, representing more than 30,000 businesses, provide HIV education. Of these, nearly all indicated that the program includes a lecture, seminar, or discussion group. Almost three-quarters of the businesses surveyed indicated that the programs were mandatory for at least some managers, supervisors, and employees.

One of the objectives of the survey was to follow up on whether businesses had adopted the CDC-sponsored "Business Responds to AIDS Workplace Program." Five core elements make up the program:

1. Businesses should develop an HIV/AIDS policy.
2. They should train supervisors in the policy.
3. They should provide HIV/AIDS education for employees.
4. They should provide HIV/AIDS education for the families of employees.
5. They should encourage employee volunteerism, community service, and corporate philanthropy.

The survey indicated that most businesses had indeed installed the program.

 ## AIDS and Medical Care

Through the early years of the AIDS epidemic, there was some question as to whether physicians, dentists, and other medical professionals could refuse to treat potentially HIV-infected people without violating state discrimination laws. That question has been resolved in various states by the state courts. For example, a ruling handed down by the New York Court of Appeals concerned a suit brought by a patient against a dentist for allegedly refusing treatment. The Court ruled that dentists' offices are "places of public accommodation" because they provide services to the public, and as such, their jurisdiction comes under the state's human rights law. The ruling sent the message to dentists, doctors, and other medical professionals that they are not exempt from human rights law.

Indeed, a study performed during the 1990s implies that the focus on the future of the AIDS epidemic rests largely with healthcare providers. The study puts the burden of dealing with the AIDS epidemic squarely on the back of the health professional: it showed that all groups progress to AIDS with equal speed, and that the unequal progression has primarily to do with unequal access to medical care. Furthermore, the study showed that the individual's social behaviors, apart from access to medical care, probably do not influence how the AIDS progresses.

The study was performed at the Johns Hopkins University School of Medicine in Baltimore, Maryland. Physicians and researchers analyzed health information from over 1300 people who attended the Johns Hopkins HIV clinic for treatment over a 5-year period. Researchers measured the individual's disease progression by noting their T cell counts. Among people with comparable initial T cell counts, the scientists found no association between survival rates or AIDS progression as they relate to race, sex, use of injection drugs, income, education, and/or insurance coverage. The study cast doubt on correlations of this type reported from other studies.

The broad range of the study in the subject pool lends weight to the idea that access to medical care predicts survival more readily than other characteristics. Some other factors did correlate with lower or higher rates of survival, but these factors were consistent with the study's findings. For example, people who had received AZT therapy before coming to the clinic or enrolling in the study had a lower rate of survival but this was presumably because they had more advanced HIV infections. In addition, older patients had lower survival rates, presumably because their bodies are less able to cope with the lower immunity to other diseases caused by HIV infection.

AIDS Spending

The current budget at the U.S. National Institutes of Health for AIDS research and education is approximately $1.5 billion. Advocacy groups seeking equal allocations for other diseases have challenged spending this relatively large amount of money on a single disease. Some groups feel that they deserve a funding allocation corresponding to the size of their patient population; for example, AIDS gets a large allocation even though the number of HIV-infected people is relatively small compared to the number who suffer from cancer.

But AIDS researchers and administrators staunchly defend the spending on AIDS research. The former head of the NIH, Harold Varmus, pointed out that AIDS is the country's leading cause of death for 25 to 44 year olds. He also argued that the disease should get special attention because a public health emergency exists so long as AIDS is new and still spreading. Furthermore, health officials reason that AIDS is caused by an identifiable virus, and history has shown that vaccines can be used against such pathogens. They point out that when resources were put into polio research, a vaccine was developed and the epidemic was halted. The same has not held true for other diseases such as cancer and diabetes.

A Vaccine for AIDS

Probably the single most important long-term goal of current research efforts is the development of an AIDS vaccine. However, a vaccine that fully prevents the establishment of HIV infection is a daunting goal. Judging from the limited progress thus far, even a vaccine that offers a significant reduction of disease and mortality appears to be a difficult task.

Producing an AIDS vaccine might appear rather straightforward: cultivate a huge batch of HIV, inactivate the viruses with chemicals, purify the preparation, and prepare it for the vaccination candidate. Unfortunately, the reality is much more complex than this. For example, a batch of bad vaccine could be deadly to its recipients—indeed, people are usually reluctant to be immunized with any whole viral particles, much less HIV particles, regardless of how inactive they are said to be. It is likewise apparent that people would not accept a vaccine composed of weakened HIV particles, as they currently accept the weakened virus in the measles vaccine. There is also the problem of the extensive mutations that take place in HIV, especially in the glycoproteins in the spikes of its envelope. Each mutant elicits a different antibody. A vaccine would have to take the potential for mutant strains into account as well.

Despite these concerns, developing an AIDS vaccine remains a major priority of researchers because in the United States alone about 20 million people would be vaccine candidates. This group would include anyone practicing high risk behaviors such as unprotected sexual intercourse, anyone using drugs, or anyone coming in contact with blood. In the latter group are such diverse individuals as surgeons, doctors, dentists, medical technologists, morticians, emergency medical technicians, firefighters, and police officers.

Modern vaccine technologists are focusing their attention on gp120 and gp41, two key glycoproteins in the HIV envelope. They have identified the genes that encode these proteins, cloned the genes, and inserted them to host yeast cells. The latter have had their biochemistry altered and have produced high volumes of gp41 and gp120 proteins for use as

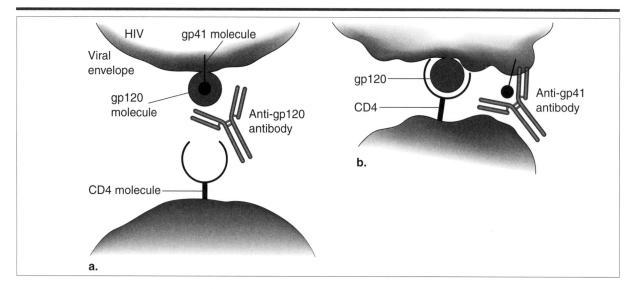

FIGURE 10.2   How an AIDS vaccine works. The union of HIV with its host T cell depends on union of the gp120 and gp41 molecules with the CD4 receptor site, the membrane of the host cell, and other coreceptors. (a) When pure gp120 molecules are injected into the body, the immune system responds with anti-gp120 antibodies. The latter circulate and when HIV enters the body, an antibody molecule reacts with the gp120 molecule thereby preventing it from uniting with the CD4 molecule. (b) Similarly, an anti-gp41 antibody prevents the gp4l molecule from reaching the host cell surface. So neutralized, the virus cannot enter its host cell and replicate. Infection is thus prevented.

immunizing agents. The theory is that, when these agents are injected into the body, the immune system will produce antibodies that react with the spikes in the HIV envelope, and prohibit the virus from reaching helper T cells. Figure 10.2 illustrates how such a vaccine might work. Tests are currently underway to determine whether these vaccines are useful.

Another potential vaccine uses a genetically engineered strain of HIV that has no envelope, the theory being that without the envelope the virus cannot enter target cells. Other researchers are concentrating on simian immunodeficiency, a virus of chimpanzees that is a close relative of HIV. They hope to use this virus in a vaccine much as a vaccine containing cowpox viruses has been used for centuries against smallpox viruses. Whether SIV could cause human disease is uncertain, however.

Numerous problems must be resolved before any of these vaccines is useful. For example, there is the question of how to reach HIV particles that have penetrated into T cells, because antibodies do not penetrate cells. An animal model for testing vaccines must also be found because chimpanzees are the only animals known to display AIDS symptoms, and chimpanzees are in very limited supply. Field trials also illustrate the problems confronting AIDS vaccine development: volunteers can only be used once, and there are various candidate vaccines available for testing. In addition, volunteers will test positive for HIV antibodies after participating in a trial; and should the volunteers acquire HIV infection, the diagnostic test for antibodies would not be useful. In addition, they might suffer discrimination in obtaining insurance or housing because their antibody test for HIV infection will be positive.

Another problem concerns counseling. When a person volunteers for a vaccine trial, the physician is ethically obliged to counsel the person on how to avoid AIDS. It would therefore be difficult to determine whether the person remained free of AIDS because of the counseling or because of the vaccine. Finally, scientists must know whether the immune response from a vaccine protects the body. If the person has developed antibodies from the vaccine, it would be unethical to inject that individual with HIV to determine whether the antibodies are protective. And these are but a few of the problems that must be circumvented.

In the United States today, approximately $1.5 billion is spent on AIDS education and research, and approximately one-half that amount is spent directly or indirectly on vaccine research. Nobel laureate David Baltimore is currently the head of the U.S. government effort to develop the vaccine. Although several companies and private charities are funding vaccine efforts as well, a promising vaccine has yet to be developed and it is unlikely that an effective immunization program will be available until the next generation.

 Social Science and AIDS

Our society is faced with the formidable challenge of reducing the fatalities associated with AIDS, even though scientists agree that a completely effective cure or vaccine for this disease is many years away. However, because scientists know that AIDS is transmitted through specific social behaviors, they believe it can be prevented by behavioral changes. Thus, society can take steps to stem the loss of human life by building on knowledge from the social sciences.

The value of the social sciences in fighting the spread of AIDS has been highlighted in numerous reports. For example, social science studies show how the power of social norms and social mores can affect prevention programs. Researchers have shown that injection drug users who understand the social rules of their group are effective in getting other drug users to adopt preventive behavior or decrease high risk activities. Researchers have also found that when drug users educate other drug users about how AIDS spreads, they share equipment less frequently, use shooting galleries less often, and decrease the number of injections they take per month. They are also more likely to take precautions such as using new needles or using bleach to sterilize their needles.

Similarly, social science researchers have shown that behavioral changes also occur when leaders in gay communities are trained to encourage safe sex practices. A study found that, after three months of peer-led AIDS education, the gay men in one community reduced their practice of unprotected sex by as much as 15 percent to 25 percent. Peer-led AIDS education may also be useful for reducing high-risk behavior among members of other groups, including sexually active teenagers and people involved in sexual relationships with injection drug users.

In another study, researchers found that 83 percent of Americans surveyed had had only one or in some cases no sexual partner during the previous year. These findings suggest that researchers should target AIDS prevention messages at the remaining 17 percent of the population who are likely to be most sexually active. In many cases the target is young, unmarried men. This approach concentrates the AIDS prevention message where it is most useful, rather than defusing the message over the entire American population.

Ethics and AIDS

Since the earliest days of the AIDS epidemic, AIDS has challenged ethical precepts and has attracted more attention from ethicists than any other disease of contemporary significance. AIDS continues to test the mettle of society and raise questions that can be ethically considered from two opposing viewpoints.

On numerous occasions, the ethics of discrimination against HIV-infected individuals has entered the picture. Discrimination in hiring and housing have been well-known practices, and the ethical question has arisen of whether insurance companies can refuse to write policies for HIV-positive individuals. As recently as 1998, the U.S. Supreme Court ruled that individuals having HIV infection and without symptoms of AIDS are protected under Americans with Disabilities Act of 1990, which bars discrimination against people with disabilities. The decision was based on the case of a woman who had sought treatment from a dentist but was rejected because the dentist feared viral transmission.

Another ethical issue concerns the cost of HIV therapy. The best available therapy, combining three drugs to suppress viral replication often costs more than $10,000 a year. Although some states have allocated funds to treat poorer individuals, the funds are limited and the poor generally have less access to treatment than those with good health insurance policies. Thus, ethics enters into the picture of how to treat all individuals with equity. Table 10.1 presents some whole costs for anti-HIV medications and drugs.

There is also the issue of complex therapy involving three drugs (Chapter 9). In many cases, eight or more pills must be taken daily in addition to other possible medications. Patients who are unable or unwilling to follow these strict regimens will discover that treatments are ineffective. Physicians therefore advise against the therapy for patients who are judged unlikely to follow the regimen. This creates the ethical dilemma of who should be treated and how.

Ethics also enters the picture during clinical trials. It has become clear that a single anti-HIV drug does not work well alone, so all clinical trials should be conducted with drug combinations. However, such an approach makes it difficult to gauge the effects of a single drug while maintaining good ethics.

Ethics continues to be a factor when rich countries such as the United States sponsor drug trials in poor countries such as African nations where the results of the drug trials could not possibly be used. For example, many studies of therapy are conducted with medicines so expensive that, were the trials to be successful, the medicine could not possibly be used in that country. AZT, for instance, has been tested as a drug for preventing passage of HIV during pregnancy, but the drug regimen during the last 26 weeks of pregnancy costs about $800—far too expensive for widespread use in developing countries. Thus, ethicists maintain that drugs should be tested only where they are potentially useful and where there is a plan at the outset to make the treatment available to the local population if it proves effective.

Ethical dilemmas also enter the picture when candidate vaccines are available for trials in HIV-infected individuals. Should the individual switch and become a candidate for the vaccine trial? Or should the patient continue to receive the drug therapy? Some ethicists maintain that the therapy must be offered to all participants in the vaccine trial, but if this is the case, then the value of the vaccine cannot be properly evaluated against the unvaccinated. It is clear that the HIV epidemic will continue to tax the conscience of society until an inexpensive effective therapy and a successful vaccine are in place for all individuals.

The Changing Landscape of AIDS

The AIDS epidemic is now devastating a different group of the American population than those initially infected. From the first appearance of AIDS in the United States in the late 1970s through the middle of the 1980s, the AIDS epidemic was concentrated in white homosexual men in major metropolitan areas such as New York, San Francisco, and Los Angeles. During the 1990s and into the 21st century, the AIDS epidemic has become increasingly concentrated among racial minorities, and it has involved more and more women, not only in cities but in rural areas, especially in the southern United States.

In addition, the epidemic is increasingly linked with illicit drugs. It is spreading among people who are inadequately constrained by social norms, including the laws pertaining to drugs (Figure 10.3). Such individuals are impervious to the aggressive dissemination of public health information, a factor that increases the burden on the public health network that is trying to reach them.

Public health officials have hoped that, because AIDS has been an epidemic driven by behavior, the epidemic can be contained by changing behavior. However, a disquieting comparison can be made to another, simpler, behavior-driven epidemic: smoking. Even though smoking involves a powerful addiction to nicotine and is related to lung cancer, all the information made available to the public has had only a slight effect in reducing the number of smokers. By contrast, the spread of AIDS is often entangled with sexual impulses and combined with heroin or cocaine addiction, drives that are even more substantial than nicotine addiction. Just as aggressive educational campaigns have not been completely successful with smoking, aggressive programs teaching about AIDS may not be the answer to interrupting the AIDS epidemic.

A Deceiving Calm

During the 1990s, a turning point in the battle against AIDS occurred with the introduction of the protease inhibitors. These drugs promised to transform what was once considered a terminal illness into a chronic, manageable condition. As the search now widened for a total cure, the environment was recharged, and people began believing that AIDS was fast becoming a disease one could live with, rather than die from.

Indeed, for those with the right body chemistry and the economic, medical, and social support necessary to succeed, the new treatment regimens mean better health, as well as increased stamina and a new lease on life. In the period of January to September 1996, the number of overall AIDS deaths not only stopped their upward climb, but fell by 19 percent.

Any drop in AIDS deaths is received as good news, but health officials cautioned that it was too early to claim victo-

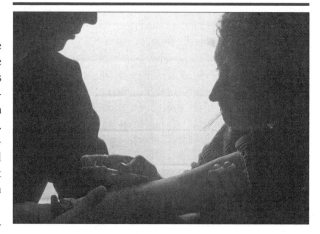

FIGURE 10.3 Injection drug users are poorly constrained by social norms and are resistant by behavioral modification programs. The upsurge of AIDS among this group is expected to be considerable in the years ahead.

ry, especially as the gains were not universal. For example, although AIDS deaths dropped by 22 percent among men, they only dropped 7 percent among women. Similarly, deaths fell by 28 percent among whites, but only 16 percent among Hispanics and only 10 percent among blacks. Furthermore, the protease inhibitors did not work for everyone, and there were many stories of those who found the drugs inaccessible, toxic, or ineffective.

The realization that AIDS has become a treatable disease for some has overshadowed the fact that AIDS is probably 100 percent preventable. The positive development that the HIV epidemic has reached a plateau is counterbalanced by the observation that the plateau is terribly high—particularly for a disease transmitted almost entirely by behaviors that have been abundantly publicized as putting people at risk. Unfortunately, the growing popular notion that living with AIDS simply means popping a few pills each day has given many individuals the license to abandon safer sex practices. Ironically, the medical advances designed to solve a public health crisis may in some ways be making that crisis worse.

In addition, some doctors are reportedly starting to use the powerful new drugs to try to prevent infection in patients who show up in their offices the morning after a night of unsafe sex. There are no studies supporting the use of protease inhibitors as preventives, but some doctors are hoping that the same drug therapy used to prevent HIV infection in healthcare workers accidentally stuck with needles can be used in those exposed to HIV by unsafe sex or other means. Some individuals have come to view the new drugs as a type of "morning-after pill." Counselors must spend hours explaining that the treatments have substantial side effects, cost several thousand dollars, and have not been proven to prevent HIV infection.

It has now become clear that the protease inhibitors have

TABLE 10.1 The Wholesale Costs of Anti-HIV Drugs and Medications, 1999

Opportunistic Pathogen	Drug	Dose	Annual Cost per Patient
Pneumocystis carinii	Trimethoprin sulfamethoxazole	160/800 mg q.d.	$60
	Dapsone	100 mg q.d.	$72
	Aerosolized pentamidine	300 mg q.m.	$1,185
	Atovaquone	1500 mg q.d.	$10,647
Mycobacterium avium complex	Clarithromycin	500 mg b.i.d.	$2,347
	Azithromycin	1,200 mg q.w.	$1,635
	Rifabutin	300 mg q.d.	$3,352
Cytomegalovirus	Ganciclovir (po)	1,000 mg t.i.d.	$17,269
	Ganciclovir implant		$5,000
	Ganciclovir (iv)	5 mg/kg q.d.	$9,113
	Foscarnet (iv)	90–120 mg/kg q.d.	$27,960–36,770
	Cidofovir (iv)	375 mg q.o.w.	$19,812
	Fomivirsen (intravitreal)	1 vial every 4 weeks	$12,000
Mycobacterium tuberculosis	Isoniazid	300 mg q.d.	$23
	Rifampin	600 mg q.d.	$1,540
	Pyrazinamide	1,500 mg q.d.	$1,005
	Ethambutol	900 mg q.d.	$1,527
Fungi	Fluconazole	200 mg q.d.	$4,267
	Itraconazole capsules	200 mg q.d.	$4,893
	Itraconozole solution	200 mg q.d.	$5,129
	Ketoconazole	200 mg q.d.	$1,230
Herpes simplex virus	Acyclovir	400 mg b.i.d.	$1,300
	Famciclovir	500 mg b.i.d.	$4,826
	Valacyclovir	500 mg b.i.d.	$1,435
Toxoplasma gondii	Pyrimethamine	50 mg q.w.	$45
	Leucovorin	25 mg q.w.	$1,248
	Sulfadiazine	500 mg q.i.d.	$1,421
Varicella zoster virus	VZIG	5 vials (6.25 ml)	$560

been a godsend for some individuals but a disappointment for others and minimally useful for prevention efforts. Unless sustained attention is devoted to prevention, HIV will destroy whatever gains have been made, and AIDS will once again prosper as have syphilis, gonorrhea, and tuberculosis, all of which have reemerged in society and thrived in part on complacency. The calm now perceived in the AIDS epidemic is not only deceptive but dangerous if it prompts health officials to relax their vigilance and lose sight of the continuing threat.

 ## The Challenges Ahead

The first two decades of AIDS research emphasized the nation's commitment to respond promptly and vigorously. During this time, scientists obtained a deep understanding of the pathogenesis of the disease. Two classes of useful drugs, the reverse transcriptase inhibitors and the protease inhibitors, have been introduced. The likelihood of transmis-

sion of HIV from a pregnant woman to her child has been remarkably diminished. Treatments for opportunistic illnesses have prolonged life and improved the quality of life for people living with AIDS.

Nonetheless, these achievements have not been accompanied by the robust therapies that were hoped for, nor is a highly effective preventive vaccine in sight. Our ability to alter risk-taking behaviors is still very limited. Scientists do not understand many aspects of HIV's interaction with the infected individual, nor do they fully understand the nature of the host response to the virus.

In the years ahead, AIDS researchers must delve deeply into several arenas. Primate research must be encouraged because it plays a role in understanding the pathogenesis of AIDS. The form of immunity most effective against HIV must be determined, and the source of protective immunity must be understood. The nature of the immunodeficiency surrounding AIDS must be more thoroughly researched. New classes of drugs giving effective chemotherapy combinations must be located. And behavioral research must be encouraged as an essential component in building the knowledge base on AIDS.

In the workplace, managers must maintain an atmosphere in which the transmission of HIV is prevented. This should be part of a general effort to maintain health and prevent industrial accidents. Further, misinformation should not lead to discrimination, and no one should lose his or her job because of false beliefs regarding AIDS transmission.

In the streets, treatment should be available for all injection drug users, with supportive therapy and psychological counseling. Many believe that bottles of bleach already diluted should be available for cleaning needles and syringes, and that inexpensive condoms should be available in vending machines accessible to all individuals. Needle distribution programs have been shown to work, and they probably should be encouraged. Governments should consider carefully supervising the health of prostitutes to control sexually transmitted diseases. Further research into the reasons for prostitution, including the low self-esteem of women and the victimization of women through exploitation, should be investigated.

Those who interact with AIDS patients should reflect society's commitment to their care and elicit their cooperation and trust. There should, for example, be no difference in the care given to a patient who has AIDS and one who has influenza. Most AIDS patients are able to live many years with their diseases, but for many a final slide toward death ensues. The hospice and home care management systems have made this time peaceful and comfortable, and they should be encouraged and developed further. Hospital administrators also deal with the fear of infection among their personnel, although these fears are based more from public hysteria than from actual numbers. Occupational accidents must be dealt with promptly and with adequate counseling. Managers of hospitals must ensure that the healthcare workers do not neglect AIDS patients, and that the workers observe standard universal precautions.

In the medical laboratory new policies should be developed for drug development. The tendency has been to relax some of the restrictions on experimental drugs and permit their use with terminal patients. News of vaccine trials continues to appear in public media, and vaccine development will take center stage for many years ahead. The spur of competition will continue to drive researchers forward until the epidemic finally subsides. In the end, education and social change can probably do as much to interrupt the AIDS epidemic as drug therapies.

The Future of AIDS

With the beginning of the 21st century, a casual browser of a recent newsstand might conclude that AIDS epidemic is all but over. Contributing to this perception are the headlines in such publications as the *New York Times Magazine*, which featured a cover story headline that read "When AIDS Ends." A late-1990s, *Newsweek* cover speculated about "The End of AIDS?". And in 1996 the cover of *Time* magazine toasted AIDS researcher David Ho as its "Man of the Year" (Figure 10.4).

To be sure, AIDS research had a banner year in 1996 when it made dramatic strides with potent new drug therapies. Indeed, *Science* magazine featured the new anti-HIV drugs as the "breakthrough of the year." But AIDS researchers are somewhat concerned that the popular media stories cross the line separating hope from hype. Even though many stories point out the shortcomings of the drugs, researchers worry that the headlines overpower the precautions. They worry that the fine print does not adequately explain that the new drugs don't work on every patient and have serious toxic side effects.

A positive note is seen in the finding released by a foundation study in early 1998. The poll indicates that while people are very optimistic about the advances made in science, they continue to be realistic about the fact that there is no cure as yet for AIDS. The foundation questioned about 2500 adults and found that 88 percent completely disagreed with

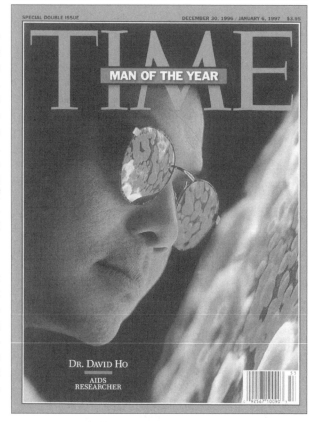

FIGURE 10.4 Headlines trumpeting the end of the AIDS epidemic are premature at this juncture. Effective cures and vaccines still await development. Until they are available, education is the key preventative measure against the spread of AIDS.

the statement that "the AIDS epidemic is over." They found that 83 percent agreed that AIDS continues to be "a major threat to public health." Moreover, the poll found that 52 percent of adults believe that the United States is making progress against AIDS (a number up from 32 percent in 1995), and 86 percent believe that "AIDS drugs can lengthen lives." And an equal number knew that the drugs for AIDS treatment are not cures for AIDS.

When the AIDS epidemic began in 1981, scientists and doctors believed that a cure or a vaccine would be available within 5 to 10 years. Few imagined that HIV would continue to plague humanity a full generation later. Today's teenagers are growing up in the Age of AIDS, and it is likely that the epidemic will continue to be a world crisis when they have their children.

According to the United Nations AIDS Programme based in Geneva, Switzerland, over 30 million people in the world live with HIV infection. Moreover, at least 90 percent of them live in the poorer countries of the world where they cannot afford the drugs available to HIV patients in the United States. In certain African countries such as Uganda, Zimbabwe, and Tanzania, more than one-third of all adults are infected with HIV; and the United Nations AIDS Programme predicts that the virus will continue to afflict those societies well into the middle of the 21st century.

In addition, world health agencies continue to express concerns for such countries as China and India, each with over a billion people. HIV is now spreading in those countries, and because of their huge populations, even a fraction of infection in the populations would be devastating. For example, if just 2 percent of the Indian population is infected with HIV by 2010, the number of infected individuals would be 20 million patients. The UN AIDS Programme estimates that about 2 million Indian citizens are already infected. For these and many other people of the world, drugs to treat HIV are unaffordable—in many sub-Saharan countries of Africa, less than $5 is spent on all healthcare needs per person each year. Unfortunately, a single pill of many HIV drugs costs more than $5. Although tremendous gains have been made in using the anti-HIV drugs in the United States, these gains have not been applied to the remainder of the world.

There is also the issue of length of treatment period. The longer people take the therapy, the more likely that the drug toxicity will become unbearable. Moreover, mutant, drug-resistant HIV particles develop in patients' bodies and overwhelm them, causing a progression to AIDS. And even when HIV is cleared from the blood, the possibility also exists that it will remain in the person's cells where the immune system cannot destroy it. New surveys in the United States indicate that 9 percent to 11 percent of all new HIV infections involve strains of the virus resistant to drugs. Taken together, these disturbing findings underscore the desperate need for an AIDS vaccine.

Still, there are the gains to be considered. For the first two decades of the AIDS epidemic, an increasing mortality rate was seen in the United States. Then, in 1998, scientists celebrated the fact that the death rate in the United States attributable to AIDS had declined significantly for the first time. It was satisfying to note that the explanation was almost entirely based on use of antiretroviral therapies. That success derived from the full disclosure of viral genes, the chemical analysis of viral dynamics and pathogenesis, and the development of protein-targeted drugs. Federal agencies and private foundations largely funded the investigator-driven basic science, and the pharmaceutical industry and biotechnology companies undertook drug discovery and development. The public and private sectors interacted to transfer knowledge and foster its application. The success of AIDS reduction mortality affirmed the vigor of this system.

Although the drugs are expensive, and there is a continued high rate of viral transmission in the United States and a growing epidemic in poorer parts of the world, scientists must pause to contemplate the success of the antiretroviral therapy. But these successes have also bred new challenges. Improved versions of current drugs must be developed. Viral variation must be better understood to help scientists cope with drug resistance. Active research programs are needed to seek new classes of compounds targeted against other viral functions, with the prospect of complementing existing drugs. And behavioral research should improve compliance with current regimens and enhance the current strategies aimed at reducing the transmission of the virus. When these challenges have been successfully met, we can anticipate an end to the AIDS epidemic—but not before.

Questions

1. Outline some unique problems associated with AIDS in women, in adolescents, in the workplace, and in the medical community.

2. Explain the components of the various AIDS vaccines being developed and summarize some pitfalls in AIDS vaccine development.

3. Discuss a number of ethical dilemmas that have developed during the course of the AIDS epidemic.

Index

Acquired immunodeficiency virus.
See AIDS; HIV infection
Acute disease, 10
Acute primary infection, 27
Acyclovir, costs of, 74, 83*t*
Adolescents, AIDS in, 78
Africa
    AIDS epidemic in, 5, 85
    drug trials in, 81
    gender distribution of AIDS
        cases in, 39
    high AIDS-related morality
        rates in, 77
    HIV-2 in, 36
    HIV-1 O group in, 21
    HIV strains in, 8
    social change in, 7
African chimpanzees, 6
African primates, 1
AIDS. *See also* HIV-1; HIV-2; HIV
        infection
    apoptosis in, 22–23
    in blood product recipients, 41
    case definition for, 29–35
    cases of reported by exposure
        category and gender, 42*t*
    changing landscape of, 82–83
    in children, 30
    denial of, 78
    diagnosing, 59–65
    distribution of in population
        groups, 38
    early observations of, 2–3
    early suspects in, 3
    emergence of, 1–7
    epidemic of, 4
        recent statistics on, 4–5
        social impact of, 76–85
        spread of, 37–43
    ethics and, 81
    first cases of, 2
    first use of term, 3
    future challenges for, 83–85
    genetic immunity to, 20
    global morality rates from, 21
    global spread of, 8
    healthcare workers and, 52–58
    HIV-2 and, 36
    versus HIV infection, 1
    as infectious disease, 3–4
    isolation and cultivation
        of virus in, 3
    medical care and, 79
    mortality rate for, 77
        declining, 82
        estimated, 5*t*
    opportunistic illnesses
        associated with, 37.
        See also Opportunistic
            illness
    pandemic of, 5
    perinatal, 35
    progression to, 29–30
    public health challenge of, 1

social science and, 80–81
spending on, 79–80
treatment of, 66–75
vaccine for. *See* Vaccines
in workplace, 79
AIDS education, 80
AIDS-indicator conditions, 29
AIDS patients
    adolescent and teen, 78
    female, 77–78
    psychological burden on, 77
    social burden on, 77
AIDS-related complex, 28–29
Americans with Disabilities Act, 81
Amphotericin B
    for AIDS-defining
        opportunistic illness, 74
    for AIDS-related fungal
        disease, 32–33
Anal intercourse
    in early AIDS cases, 2
    HIV-1 B subtype
        transmission through, 41
    in HIV transmission, 39, 44
Anatomical barriers, 10
Angiographic procedures, 56
Animalborne pathogens,
    avoidance of, 49–50
Anonymous testing, 65
Anti-HIV antibodies, 59, 71
    detection of, 62
Anti-HIV drugs
    costs of, 8, 48, 83*t*, 85
    public knowledge about,
        84–85
Anti-HIV immune response,
    64–65
Antibodies, 3, 9
    mechanisms of, 14*f*
    production of, 12, 14
Antibody-mediated immunity,
    11, 13f, 37
Antibody tests, 60–62, 76
Antifungal agents, 74
Antigen-bearing macrophage, 12
Antigens, 11, 13*f*
    release of, 12
Antiretroviral drugs
    improved versions of, 85
    prophylactic, 57–58
Antiretroviral therapy, 30
    benefits and risks of, 72*t*
    CDC principles of, 67*t*
    methods of, 76
    for pediatric HIV, 73
    practical considerations in, 70
    in restoration of immune
        system, 74–75
Antiseptics, postexposure, 57
Antiviral drugs, 67
Apoptosis, 22–23, 27
Asymptomatic infection period, 27
Atovaquone, costs of, 83*t*

Azidothymidine (AZT), 4, 8, 65,
        67–68, 76
    cost of, 81
    mechanism of action of, 68*f*, 69*t*
    for mother-to-infant
        transmission, 52
    for pediatric HIV, 72–73
    for perinatal AIDS
        prevention, 35
    in postexposure prophylaxis,
        57–58
    during pregnancy, 59
    prenatal use of, 48
Azithromycin
    for AIDS-defining
        opportunistic illness, 74
    costs of, 83*t*

B cells, 11, 15, 25
    in immunity, 11–14
    production of, 13*f*
Bacterial infections
    AIDS-related, 33
    pathogenicity of, 9
Bacterial vaginosis, 40
Baltimore, David, 80
Bartonella infection, 50, 52
    animalborne, 49
Behavioral changes, in AIDS
    prevention, 80–81
Belgian Congo, polio vaccination
    campaigns in, 6
Berger, Edward, 20
Bisexual men, female sex
    partners of, 2–3
Bloodborne pathogens
    standards, 58
Bloodborne transmission, 8
Blood-brain barrier, HIV
    transport across, 34
Blood precautions, universal, 56–57
Blood products
    contamination of, 44
    recipients of, 41
    safety in handling, 48
Blood supply, safety of, 50–51
Blood tests, 4
Blood-to-blood transmission, 41, 44
Blood transfusions, 44
    HIV transmission from, 41
    recipients of, 2
Body fluids
    healthcare workers'
        exposure to, 55
    safety in handling, 48
    universal precautions
        with, 56–57
Bone marrow, B cells in, 12
Brain, immune system influence
    on, 34–35
Brazil, HIV-2 in, 36
Breast-feeding, HIV transmission
    through, 43, 44
Budding, 18

"Business Responds to AIDS
    Workplace Program" (CDC), 79

Cameroon, HIV-1 O group in, 21
Campylobacteriosis
    animalborne, 49
    prevention of, 48–49
Cancers, AIDS-related, 29t, 34
    mortality rate for, 34
Candida albicans, 29, 37
    AIDS-related, 32
        electron micrograph of, 33*f*
        treatment of, 74
Candidiasis
    with HIV-2 infection, 36
    oral, in male homosexual, 2
Capsid, 16
Capsid proteins, 18
Capsomeres, 16
    synthesis of, 18
Cardiac catheterization,
    precautions for, 56
Castanospermine, 71
Casual contact, 43
Cat scratch fever, 49, 50
Cats, pathogens transmitted by,
    49–50
CC-CKR-5 gene mutations, 20–21
CC-CKR-5 protein, 20–21
CD4, soluble, 71
CD4+ cells, 25.
    See also Helper T cells
CD8 cells, 20
CD4 proteins, 17
CD4 receptors, 17
    gp120 at, 19
    HIV binding to, 21*f*
    HIV binding to surface protein
        of, 19–20
CD26 receptors, 19–20
Cell cultures, 22
Cell death, mechanisms of, 22–23
Cell-mediated immunity, 11, 12,
    13f, 37
Cell pathologies, 25
Cell receptors, HIV and, 19–20
Cell-virus fusion, 20
Centers for Disease Control
    and Prevention (CDC)
    antiretroviral therapy
        principles of, 67t
    "Business Responds to AIDS
        Workplace Program," 79
    classification system of, 28t
    data on AIDS epidemic, 38
    Gottlieb's report to, 2
    recent AIDS statistics of, 4–5
Cesarean delivery, precautions
    for, 56
Chain terminator, 68
Chancroid, 40
Chemokine receptors, 20–21
Chemokines, 12
Chemotherapy, 71
    candidiasis with, 2

Credits

CHAPTER 1, p. 2: AP/Wide World; p. 3 left: Bob Crandall/TimePix; p. 3 right: Barbara Ries/Liaison Agency; p. 7: Courtesy of Dr. Paul Ewald. Data for tables 1.1 and 1.2 from *HIV/AIDS Surveillance Report*, Vol. 11, No. 1, June 1999.

CHAPTER 2, p. 10: David Scharf/Peter Arnold; p. 11: Microworks/PhotoTake.

CHAPTER 3, p. 23 a & b: K. Nagashima/NCI.

CHAPTER 4, p. 33 top: David Scharf/Peter Arnold; p. 33 bottom: Larry Jensen/Visuals Unlimited; p. 34: Zeva Oelbaum/Peter Arnold. Data for table 4.2 from *Morbidity and Mortality Weekly Report*, Vol. 41, RR-17, December 18, 1992. Data for table 4.5 from *Morbidity and Mortality Weekly Report*, Vol. 48, SS-2, April 16, 1999. Data for table 4.6 from *Morbidity and Mortality Weekly Report*, Vol. 48, SS-2, March 3, 1999.

CHAPTER 5, p. 39: SIU/Visuals Unlimited; p. 42: David Boe/©Bettmann/CORBIS. Data for tables 5.1 and 5.2 from *HIV/AIDS Surveillance Report*, Vol. 11, No. 1, June 1999.

CHAPTER 6, p. 47: Matt Sumner/From the Hip/The Image Works; p. 49: M. Abbey/Visuals Unlimited.

CHAPTER 7: Data for table 7.1 from *HIV/AIDS Surveillance Report*, Vol. 11, No. 1, June 1999. Data for table 7.2 courtesy of the Centers for Disease Control and Prevention.

CHAPTER 9: Data for tables 9.1, 9.2, and 9.3 from *Morbidity and Mortality Weekly Report*, Vol. 47, RR-5, April 24, 1998; data for table 9.4 from *Morbidity and Mortality Weekly Report*, Vol. 48, RR-10, August 20, 1999.

CHAPTER 10, p. 77: AP/Wide World; p. 84: Custom Medical Stock; p. 84: ©1996 Time. All rights reserved. Reprinted by permission. Data for table 10.1 from *Morbidity and Mortality Weekly Report*, Vol. 48, RR-10, August 20, 1999.